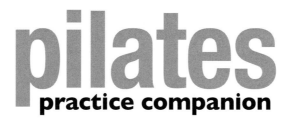

pilates
practice companion

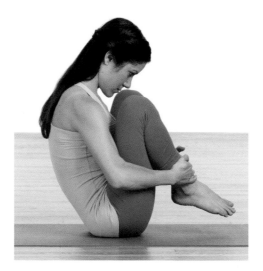

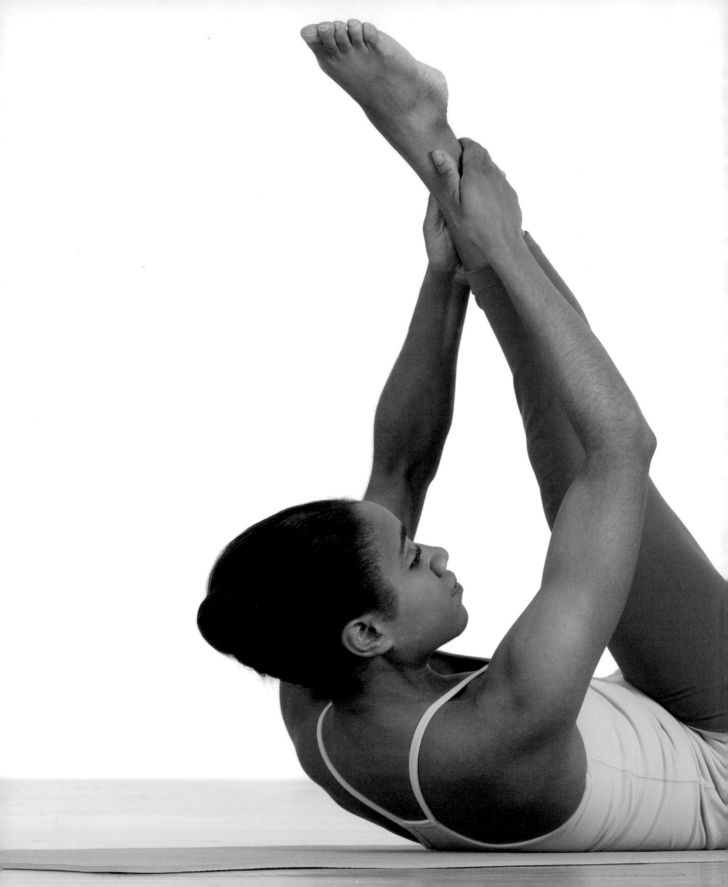

pilates
practice companion

Alycea Ungaro

London • New York • Melbourne • Munich • Delhi

Project editor Hilary Mandleberg
Designer Anne Fisher
Senior editor Helen Murray
Senior art editor Wendy Bartlet
Managing editor Penny Warren
Managing art editor Glenda Fisher
Production editor Maria Elia
Production controller Alice Sykes
Creative technical support Sonia Charbonnier
Category publisher Peggy Vance

Photographer Angela Coppola
Illustrations Peter Bull Arts Studio

First published in Great Britain in 2011 by Dorling
Kindersley Limited, 80 Strand, London, WC2R 0RL
Penguin Group (UK)

2 4 6 8 10 9 7 5 3 1

Health warning
All participants in fitness activities must assume the
responsibility for their own actions and safety. If you
have any health problems or medical conditions,
consult with your physician before undertaking any
of the activities set out in this book. The information
contained in this book cannot replace sound
judgment and good decision making, which can
help reduce risk of injury.

A CIP catalogue of this book is available from
the British Library

ISBN 978-1-4053-6038-8

Colour reproduction by Alta Image, London
Printed and bound by TWP in Singapore

Discover more at
www.dk.com

Contents

Introduction   6

The story of Pilates • The evolution of Pilates
• Pilates myths

The benefits of Pilates   14

Why do Pilates? • Breath • Proper alignment
• Strength • Stability • Flexibility • Body
control • Body shape and tone • Endurance
• Mind over muscle • Stress reduction

Before you begin   38

Learning the basics • The Six Pilates principles
• Pilates Qs and As • Clothing and equipment

The exercises   54

How this book works • Warm-Up • Beginner
level • Beginner sequences • Intermediate level
• Intermediate sequences • Advanced level
• Advanced sequences • Troubleshooting
• Joining a class

Pilates every day   218

From workout to daily life • Know your body
• Maintaining good posture • Pilates for sport
and play • Pilates at the office • Pilates for
relaxation • Pilates for better sex • Maturing
with Pilates • Pilates for rehabilitation
• The Pilates diet

Resources   250
Index   252
Acknowledgments   256

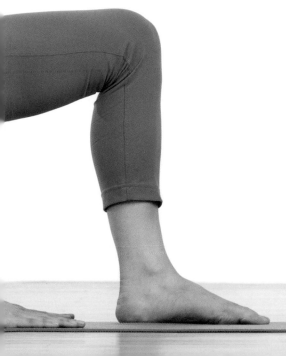

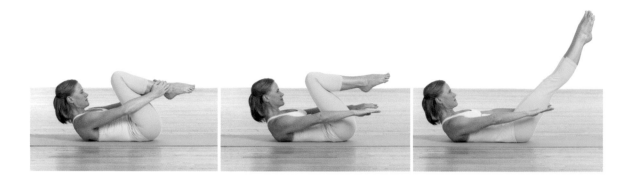

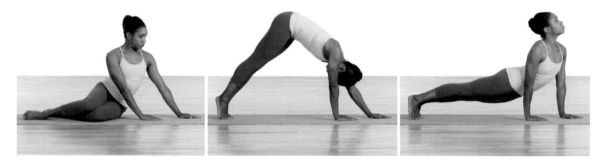

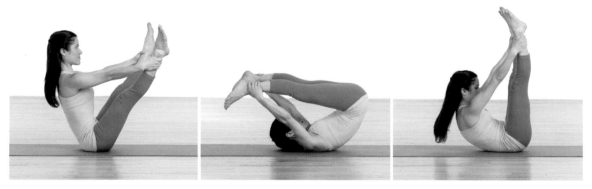

Introduction

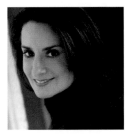

Teaching is an evolving process. Ten years have passed since I wrote my first Pilates book and for me everything has changed. While the method remains constant in its results and choreography, I can confidently say that each exercise in this book was written with new cueing and new mechanics, not because I wanted to be fresh and innovative, but because this is the way I teach today.

Since my last Pilates title, I have embraced the silent moments in teaching. My instructions have become more and more truncated and I continue to try to emphasise what I refer to as the "essence of the movement" simply with the tone of my voice. It is my sincerest wish that my tone reaches you, the reader, from the pages of this book. As much as it is possible, "listen" to the instructions. Find the accents and dynamics within each move and infuse them into your workout. These are the details that separate a run-of-the-mill exercise experience from a truly satisfying full-body workout.

Each day that I connect with a student, I discover a new word, tempo or image that changes the experience for that person, regardless of how long they have been practising Pilates. As you work through these programmes, you'll find familiar material delivered in a new way. Some exercises are in a slightly different order. Some have been crafted with a unique tempo or a modified setup. My goal is not creativity but success. Your success. As they say, there are no bad students.

Pilates is, as any training should be, personal. It should be modified to the body and to the mind so that it is the most effective training regime possible. A clever trainer must constantly adapt to the student. Using this book, become your own trainer. Adapt the work to your needs and your needs to the work. It is an honour to be able to move your body in a healthy, joyful way.

May the privilege of wellness always be yours.

The story of Pilates

What I'm about to tell you is mostly hearsay. Even as I write, several experts are trying to piece together an accurate history of Joseph Pilates, the man who invented the unique system of physical conditioning originally known as Contrology and now known the world over simply as Pilates.

The specific details and timeline of the life of Joseph Pilates are a bit of a mystery. We do know this much, though.

Joseph Pilates, also known as Joe or Uncle Joe, was born in 1883 in Mönchengladbach in Germany and was of Greek descent. His father had been a gymnast and this clearly influenced the young boy. Joe became obsessed with the Greek ideals of physical beauty and strength. He set about becoming an accomplished gymnast, like his father, as well as a diver and boxer.

Joe's career before his move to the United States was diverse. He called himself a circus performer and also worked as an anatomical model at times. His travels took him to England where he was interned when World War I broke out. Legend has it that the bulk of his exercise techniques were developed there when he worked with the other internees as well as with the patients in the camp hospital. Springs from the hospital beds were employed to create a rehabilitation programme and speed health and healing. With Germany in deep economic depression after the war, Joe Pilates chose to travel to America where many more opportunities were possible.

"In 10 sessions you will feel the difference. In 20 sessions you will see the difference. And in 30 sessions you will have a brand new body."

Joseph Pilates

The contemporary fitness scene

The exercise culture of Pilates' time was an active one. A host of "strong men" and "professors" of physical culture were on the fitness scene at the time that Joe Pilates was developing his own ideas and concepts. Eugen Sandow, Adrian Schmidt and Alex Whitely were all prolific in their methodologies and publications. Exercise devices for the home user were rapidly being created and promoted. Clearly influenced by this community, Joe Pilates set about launching his own system and his own equipment line, which incorporated the use of spring-driven resistance.

Pilates came to the United States for the first time in 1925. At that point, he was already meeting with patent lawyers to develop his unique apparatus. Some of these patents are recognisable as the Pilates apparatuses that we know today, but there are others that were either never developed or never widely utilised. Pilates was a prolific inventor.

Pilates made a second trip to America in 1926, this time to set up shop and begin building his name and reputation. According to his students at the time, his wife Clara, whom he had met on the boat to America, had the true gift of communication. Joe would create the moves, but Clara would teach them, gently nurturing the students as she taught.

The Pilates marketing machine

Mr Pilates' studio just happened to be housed in the same building as a number of dance studios. Naturally, the dancers flocked to learn the method and they were soon followed by many other devotees.

I once heard it said that Joe would turn people away when they phoned him in the early days. "No, no," he'd say brusquely. "Can't fit you in. Too busy. Call back next week." This was all part of his clever marketing plan. By giving his gym a certain cachet, he was able to draw in the opera divas, actresses and other celebrities who would go on to sing the praises of his work.

Joe Pilates also used the power of the written word to spread his message. He authored two books: the first was called *Your Health* (1934) and was a lengthy commentary on the state of civilization and how it "impairs physical fitness". The second was *Return to Life through Contrology* (1945), a home user's guide to his exercise system, in which he presented his 34 original mat exercises (see p.50).

In *Your Health*, Pilates rails at our habits, our clothes, our medical choices and even the construction of our furniture, blaming these things for all the ills of mankind.

These books weren't his only attempts at marketing. As well as his gym and his writings, Joe Pilates continued to develop exercise equipment and even dabbled in home furnishings, promoting a unique type of bed that was designed to aid healthy and natural sleep. And if you happen to watch the promotional video footage he made during the early 1930s and 1940s, you'll see how it's a portent of the sort of exercise infomercials we see today.

During the time when Joe and Clara ran their studio in New York, a select group of their most dedicated students went on to open their own studios. A handful of these fitness pioneers dedicated their lives to the teaching of the method. They were the first generation of Pilates teachers and have come to be known as the Pilates Elders. Each of them is credited with spreading the work of Joe Pilates beyond New York City and, eventually, to the world. Every teacher today can trace his or her lineage back to one of those first-generation teachers.

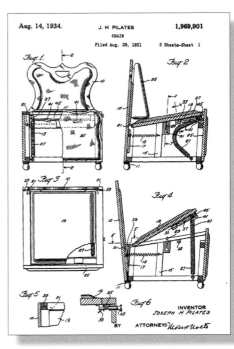

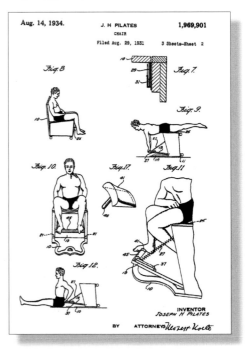

JOE PILATES' PATENT APPLICATION
Above all, Joseph Pilates was an inventor. The drawings from his patent application for a home-exercise chair illustrate his use of spring tension for muscle training.

The evolution of Pilates

To hear it said, you'd think that the Pilates method just arrived on the scene and was embraced by millions of people immediately. Although it has enjoyed a steady growth since its inception, it hasn't always been the mainstay of fitness that it is today.

The original style of Pilates that Joe taught was a forceful method of training. He was interested in visibly changing people's bodies and he didn't approach his students either slowly or gently. But as his client list grew, so did the needs of those clients. Inevitably, some clients were less capable, while others needed more care as well as modified exercises. Always the inventor, Joe Pilates' body of material grew as the needs of his students dictated.

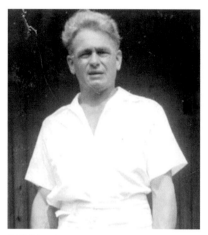

OUR FOUNDING FATHER
Joseph Hubertus Pilates, pictured here, is the father of the Pilates method that we know today.

Training the teachers

Becoming a teacher of Contrology (see p.9) in those days was by apprenticeship only. As students turned into teachers, each one of them taught the method as they had learned it. Specifically, as they had learned it for their own bodies. So, a teacher with a weak knee might know a whole repertoire of movements to strengthen the knee, while another teacher with a tight back might have learned a variety of stretching moves for the spine. Still others would have learned a series of breathing exercises.

Since there was no formalised training programme, the list of exercises taught by the instructors of that time was wildly inconsistent. Then those teachers went on to teach their students, some of whom became teachers themselves. You can imagine what the result was. Decades after Joe's death, when Pilates training programmes began to be formalised, there was no real consensus about which exercises were verifiably traceable to Joe Pilates.

The history was so rich and had been interpreted by so many people that splinters began to appear in the community. Over time, certain styles of Pilates developed as strongly therapeutic and others as more athletic. Today there exists a broad spectrum of Pilates approaches.

Pilates for everybody

I routinely answer emails and telephone calls from people wondering if Pilates is right for them. "Where should I study?" they want to know and I answer with another question, "What brought you to Pilates?" If you're looking to work out safely with scoliosis, I may recommend a slower-paced approach for you. If, on the other hand, you're training for a triathlon and want to work on your core strength, I'll recommend Pilates that is fast and furious. There is no such thing as bad Pilates – only the Pilates that is right for your body. I always say "some Pilates is better than no Pilates".

Pilates studios and classes are everywhere. They exist both independently and within mainstream health clubs. There are corporate Pilates chains and even Pilates franchises. Pilates classes stand alone but are also often combined with other disciplines, creating a Pilates–fusion workout. It's a testament to the method's effectiveness that it has not only survived but managed to thrive, no matter what the current trends in fitness may be. Pilates is truly timeless!

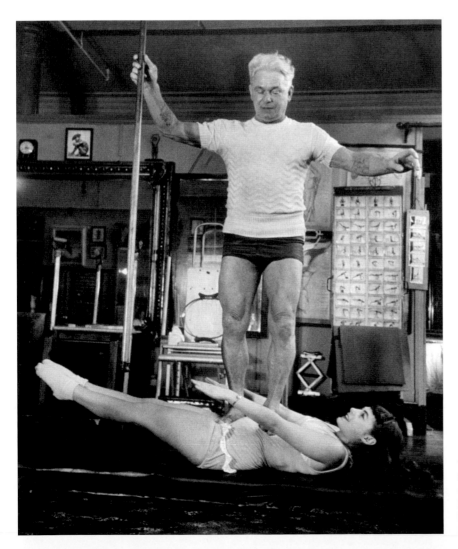

TAKE A BREATH!
Famed opera diva Roberta Peters learned a thing or two about breathing from Joe Pilates. In this picture, featured in a 1951 issue of *Life Magazine*, Peters demonstrates her warm-up exercise – The Hundred.

Pilates myths

Misconceptions abound about Pilates. Potential new students are filled with questions. They often ask for clarification about our "stretching programme" or the strange "Pilates–yoga" classes we offer. Because Pilates lacks standardisation, there's no real way to convey any universal truths about it. However, the origins of Pilates are factual. Here are the facts to counter some of those Pilates misconceptions.

"Pilates is the same as yoga."

Joe Pilates drew on many different disciplines to create his work. While Pilates is clearly influenced by certain yoga moves, the structure of the Pilates system and the focus on the physical elements, as opposed to yoga's spiritual focus, separate Pilates entirely from yoga. There's no chanting in Pilates. Nor is there any meditation. In fact, a full advanced Pilates programme bears a much stronger resemblance to calisthenics – a bodyweight system of exercises such as squats, lunges, push-ups and pull-ups that originated in Ancient Greece – than it does to yoga.

"Pilates is for dancers."

This is my favourite myth, by far. When Joe Pilates established his studio on Eighth Avenue in New York City, he was setting up shop in the same building as several dance and rehearsal studios. The influx of dancers and Joe's resulting association with dance luminaries such as George Balanchine, Martha Graham and Ted Shawn gave rise to the impression that Pilates was strictly for dancers. In fact, it was Joe Pilates' intention that his method be practised by everyone, even by schoolchildren.

"Mr Pilates was a dancer."

This idea goes hand in hand with the myth discussed above that Pilates is for dancers. No, Joe Pilates wasn't a dancer. He was a bit of a gymnast, he was part-diver part-boxer and he was an all-round fitness expert, but he was never a dancer.

"Pilates is a stretching technique."

This is true … and also not true. Here's the reality: Pilates is uniquely adaptable and as a result, every session or class can be tailored to the individual needs of the person or group. Pilates moves were created to address total fitness. Each exercise has a strength component as well as a flexibility component. If you need more strength than stretch, simply focus on that. For a more intense flexibility programme, you can gear the workout to concentrate on the stretching aspect of Pilates.

"It's great that Pilates is a no-sweat workout."

When did sweating get such a bad name? Sweating is a natural human function and a sure-fire sign that your body's burning calories. The fact is, you'll most certainly sweat in Pilates if you practise hard and move at the prescribed tempo. If you rest for long stretches in between moves, you may not get your heart rate up high enough to start sweating. At the beginning of your practice, when you're just learning the basic moves, you'll most definitely not burn hundreds of calories, but as you progress, a steady perspiration is to be expected and is appropriate.

"You always have to use machines in Pilates."

Absolutely not. In its first incarnation, Pilates consisted of floor exercises. Experimentation with springs followed and then full-on equipment (see p.8). Advanced Pilates students know full well that working on the mat is the routine you always come back to. We always say it's the "base of the method" but it's also the "crown of the method".

"Pilates is a type of physical therapy."

Actually, Pilates referred to his system as "corrective exercise". Although many argue that it's therapeutic by definition, it wasn't created solely for the purpose of physical rehabilitation. General conditioning was the goal of the method and if a bad knee got stronger or a postural misalignment improved along the way, well, so much the better.

"Pilates is a woman's exercise."

Now that's just silly. Joe Pilates was a man. He began his fitness journey training his own body and then the bodies of other men. When he was interned in England (see p.8), he trained the other interns, who were mostly men. If you watch the archival videos of Mr Pilates teaching, you'll see that he was neither gentle nor feminine in his approach. Nor was his equipment at all feminine, either in construction or appearance. I imagine Joe envisaged his gyms full of muscle-bound men toiling away as they used his springs. In truth, the Pilates system works equally well for men and women.

"Pilates is a breathing method."

This is another yes and no answer. Pilates has a full complement of breathing exercises and, while many instructors believe that the breathing techniques are vital to the practice of Pilates, some instructors never teach the breathing at all. And yet others opt to teach it only to students who are at an advanced level in their practice. Depending on your own lung capacity and cardiovascular health, your teacher will decide how much to focus on breath control during your training.

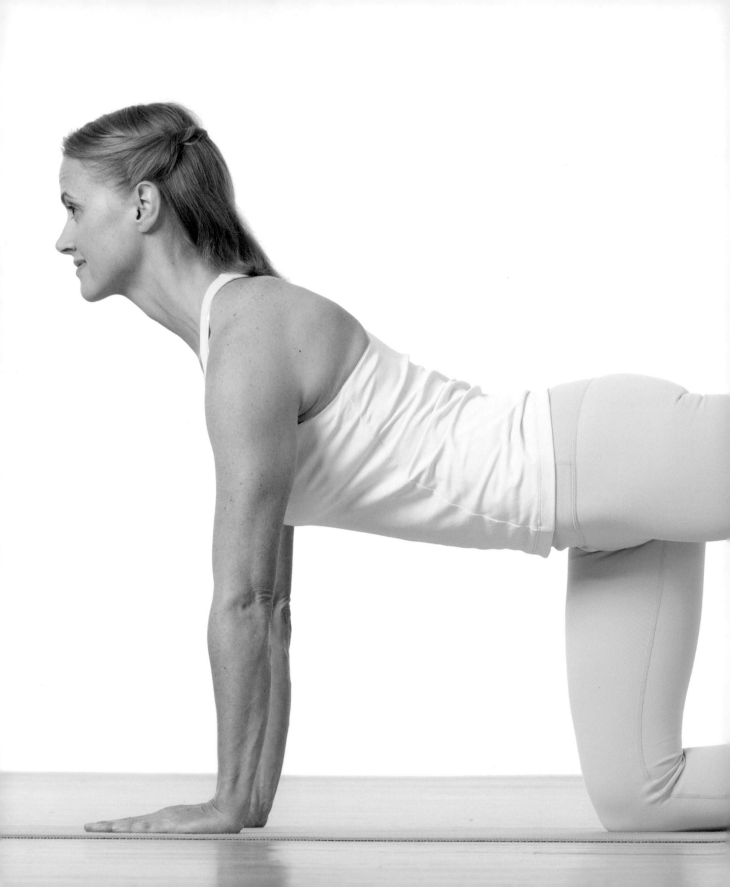

The Benefits of Pilates

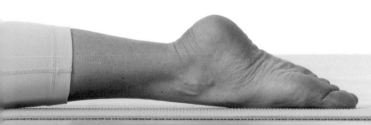

Why do Pilates?

Children play and as they do so, they exercise. Athletes compete and simultaneously train and condition their bodies. For the rest of us, the inspiration to exercise can be tough to find. In Pilates, you'll discover a training system that combines playful yet challenging movements with a competitive element that makes your exercise time truly enjoyable. Add to that the remarkable list of Pilates benefits and you've got yourself a fitness solution for life. Pilates is cross-training for real life.

You don't need me to tell you that exercise is good for you. You already know that. But in case you weren't already convinced, here are some alarming statistics you should be aware of:

- Your risk of a stroke is cut by 60% if you exercise.
- Physical activity cuts the risk of breast cancer by almost one-third.
- The risk of all forms of cancer is cut by at least 25% and the risk of death from heart disease is cut by 50% simply by engaging in regular activity.

But why should you choose Pilates rather than another type of physical activity? Pilates offers the same fundamental benefits that you can get from other sorts of training: greater body strength, improved muscle tone and more stamina are just a few. But Pilates also offers additional, less obvious benefits. Your breathing will improve, you'll become better coordinated and better aligned, your balance and stability will improve, your movements will become more graceful and easier, you'll be more flexible and your stress levels will go down. Pilates is truly magic.

Become your own teacher

This book will show you how to do Pilates and if you're already a Pilates practitioner, you'll learn how to do even better Pilates. As you read about the myriad benefits of Pilates (see box, opposite) in this chapter, you'll see that I've included some "Watchword" lists and "What's your baseline?" self-tests (see below). These simple mechanisms will help you become your own teacher as you work your way through the exercises and programmes.

WATCHWORDS! act as cues that signal your brain to focus on a specific benefit as you're doing an exercise. You'll soon become familiar with these Watchwords as you'll find them repeated throughout the exercise instructions.

"The man who uses intelligence with respect to his diet, his sleeping habits and who exercises properly, is beyond any question of doubt taking the very best preventive medicines provided so freely and abundantly by nature."

Joseph Pilates

WHAT'S YOUR BASELINE? You should do these simple self-tests before you begin. The results will give you an idea of your starting level. Every six weeks that you do your Pilates practice, check back in with your baseline measurements to see where you're making the most progress and where you still have work to accomplish.

If you're coming to Pilates to address a specific physical concern like flexibility or muscle tone, Pilates puts a wonderful tool at your disposal. The good news is all the other benefits of Pilates are included at no extra charge.

Let's get started! No matter what reason brought you to Pilates, you'll take away a host of other skills and talents.

The benefits of Pilates

A comprehensive list of the 10 key benefits of Pilates:

- Breath
- Proper alignment
- Strength
- Stability
- Flexibility
- Body control
- Body shape and tone
- Endurance
- Mind over muscle
- Stress reduction

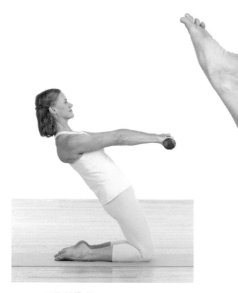

CROSS-TRAINING FOR REAL LIFE
Pilates develops strength, control and concentration.

INSIDE OUT AND UPSIDE DOWN
Using moves that work all three planes of the body, Pilates trains it from dozens of different angles to benefit every single part.

Breath

Focused and coordinated breathing is an integral part of the Pilates system. There are some simple rules and guidelines for how to breathe during Pilates. The benefits of improving your breath control go far beyond exercise.

Joe Pilates suffered from asthma as a boy. Having struggled with his own breathing, it's only logical that he would later develop an exercise system with a strong focus on breath control. One of Mr Pilates' disciples often speaks of his heavy German accent. "Brreeeeze …" he would say to his exercising pupils when instructing them to breathe out fully. Students in the room must have exhaled audibly in unison as Mr Pilates delivered his passionate instruction, training his students to empty their lungs to the maximum.

Despite his own asthma, it's often said that Mr Pilates would regularly take a jog through New York City in the dead of winter. He wore little other than his trademark white gym trunks, often seen in photos as he posed proudly in the snow. He lived to the ripe old age of 87 and was remarkably healthy all his life. There's something both tragic and ironic in the fact that advanced emphysema ultimately claimed his life.

In Pilates classes today, breath control is taught in a variety of distinct ways. Instructors agree that there's a coordination of breath and movement that exists in all Pilates workouts, but those details vary from teacher to teacher.

The benefits of coordinated breath

Here are just a few of the things you can expect simply by training your breath to coordinate with your movements:
• Increased lung capacity, which will give you better overall heart and lung (cardiopulmonary) health.
• An increase in energy and efficiency. This means you'll do more and feel less exhausted doing it.
• An increased resistance to lung-related illnesses, thanks to the improvement in the blood circulation through your heart and lungs.
• A reduction in your blood pressure.
• Better flexibility and mobility of your rib cage and spine as these bones benefit from better blood circulation.
• A greater ability to relax when you're dealing with stressful situations.

Watchwords!

Watch out for these words and phrases as you progress through the exercises in this book. They'll remind you to focus on your breathing.

• In with the air
• Wring out the lungs
• Exhale
• Expel the air
• Out through the mouth

What's your baseline?

Follow these steps to discover how well your lungs are working as you progress through the exercises in this book.

• Grab a stopwatch or watch the second hand on your clock.
• Take a deep breath in and extend it as long as you can until you can't take in any more air. Record how many seconds you can keep inhaling.
• Now wait a few moments, restore your breathing, then measure your exhalation. Breathe in to begin, then exhale slowly and steadily for as long as you can until you feel there's no more air in your lungs. Record your time.
• Repeat the inhalation and exhalation tests after you've been doing Pilates regularly for six weeks. Compare your new timings with the old ones.

"Lazy breathing converts the lungs, figuratively speaking, into a cemetery for the deposition of diseased, dying and dead germs as well as supplying an ideal haven for the multiplication of other harmful germs." Joseph Pilates

UNIQUE BREATHING STYLES

Each individual breathes in a unique way, using their skeletal and muscular structure according to their habits and training. The anatomy of respiration involves the muscles and bones, as well as the lungs themselves.

The collar bones, or clavicles, are often involved in what is known as apical or "high" breathing. In this style of breathing, the collar bones lift, raising the shoulders and pulling the abdominals inwards.

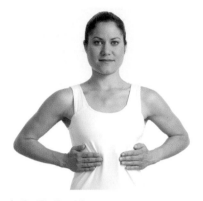

OUT WITH THE AIR

Place the hands on the ribs and exhale completely, narrowing the rib cage and helping you exhale longer.

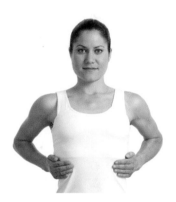

IN WITH THE AIR

Keeping your hands on your rib cage, feel how your inhalation expands your ribs from side to side and fills up the back of your body.

During respiration, the twelve pairs of ribs are moved by the intercostal muscles.

The muscles surrounding the rib cage allow the lungs to expand during inhalation. This creates a vacuum, forcing air to rush in.

Proper alignment

A well-aligned body is defined by its ability to react to all the forces around it. The most notable force acting on our bodies is gravity. Although we hardly ever acknowledge it, gravity works against us all day long. Good alignment helps minimise the impact of gravity on your body.

The neck should maintain its natural curves.

The abdominals should be pulled inwards and upwards.

The legs should be straight but not locked.

In his book *Your Health*, Pilates wrote, "practically all human ailments are directly traceable to wrong habits which can only be corrected through the immediate adoption of right (natural, normal) habits". Modern osteopaths would agree that most musculoskeletal injuries and ailments are the result of these "wrong habits" that cause imbalances and malalignments. Your body is pretty clever at compensating to avoid exertion, protect its weaknesses and exploit its strengths. But this compensation doesn't do you any favours. It just exacerbates the problems already there.

Proper alignment is something you can see simply by looking in the mirror. But it isn't just how you look from the front. It's three-dimensional. Your body should be even from side to side, front to back and top to bottom. As you exercise, you must always be aware of your alignment. Your workout is an opportunity to self-correct your malalignments. By learning to strengthen your weaknesses and correct your poor habits, you can restore optimal alignment to your body. And good alignment will ensure that you reap certain benefits such as:

- Improved posture
- More efficient mobility
- Pain-free range of motion
- Improved circulation
- Healthier organ function due to reduced organ compression.

ALIGNMENT IN PROFILE
Good alignment can be assessed by dropping a plumb line through the centre of the body in profile. The line should fall from the middle of the ear down through the shoulder and should fall slightly behind the hip joint before landing just in front of the ankle joint.

Checking your alignment

It's very easy to lose sight of staying well aligned as you exercise, but a haphazard approach will simply reinforce all of your asymmetries, preserving your weaknesses and imbalances. Muscular balance and skeletal alignment are the keys to overall "vitality" as Uncle Joe used to say. And with a bit of careful attention, this vitality can be yours.

You have two remarkable tools for checking and re-checking your alignment. The first is a mirror. Whenever possible, work out in front of a mirror. What feels balanced and even to your body may well not be. Make your workout visual. Train your eyes to train your body and your alignment will rapidly improve.

The second tool to make good use of is your exercise mat. Use it as a frame for your body. The edges of your mat will serve as a perfect grid. Whenever possible, be sure that you can see your body parts equidistant from the edges of your mat. And for most exercises, you'll want to work in the centre of the mat. Get used to gauging the distance between yourself and the sides of the mat and be sure to keep that distance equal as you move through different exercises.

One final recommendation is that you choose clothes with stitching or seams that are straight and symmetrical to help you monitor your alignment. Vertical and horizontal lines can help create an additional grid-like reference for you while you exercise. Diagonal stitching can confuse you visually so I generally avoid it.

The head should be directly in the centre of the body.

The shoulders should be level.

The weight should be balanced between each leg.

ALIGNMENT FACE ON
Pilates helps you develop muscular symmetry between the two sides of your body.

Watchwords!

Watch for these words and phrases as you progress through the exercises in this book. They'll remind you to focus on your alignment.

• Stand tall and straight

• Square your box (see p.57)

• Work within your frame (see p.57)

• Shoulders over hips

• One long line

What's your baseline?

Test your alignment with the following activity.

• Grab a camera and have a few photos taken front, side and back. Print them, then draw grid lines over the photos.

• Note if one shoulder's higher, or one hip's lower, or if your back is curved one way or the other.

• Repeat again in six weeks and compare your new photos with the old ones.

Strength

Pilates has a unique ability to make your body stronger.
With regular practice you'll not only feel, but also see,
your strength increasing.

We define strength as the ability of a muscle to do work or generate force.
Mostly, the force is produced by a muscle in response to an outside element
such as resistance. This resistance depends on the type of exercise you
practise. In Pilates we focus on two types of resistance to increase strength.
The first is the body's own weight. The second is the metal springs utilised
to construct the Pilates equipment (see p.217). The programmes in this book
are devoted to the use of your body's own weight to create resistance and
thereby strength.

As you move through your Pilates exercises, the resistance created tells
your nervous system to signal your muscle fibres to contract. This contraction
actually causes injury to the muscle by tearing the fibres. But because our
bodies are smart and adept at self-healing, the repair begins within minutes.
The muscle builds up new fibres and in the process becomes slightly bigger
than it was before. This process, known as myofibrillar hypertrophy, is
synonymous with an increase in strength. The wonderful thing about adding
muscle fibres to your body composition is that the lean body mass you're
creating makes fat that much harder to accrue.

There are many benefits to having strong muscles. Here are just a few:
• Strong muscles also mean strong ligaments and tendons, making you less
likely to injure yourself.
• Hypertrophy costs the body a lot of calories to maintain. Your body will
burn more fat simply by being stronger and leaner.
• You'll benefit from a reduction in blood pressure and improve your
cholesterol levels.
• You'll improve your balance and ability to carry out
everyday activities.

Watchwords!

Watch for these words and phrases
as you progress through the
exercises in this book. They'll
remind you to focus on the work
and strength of your muscles.

• Contract
• Tighten
• Compress
• Tense
• Squeeze

How Pilates builds strength

Pilates is a form of low-intensity resistance training. This means that no heavy weights are used. You may wonder how you'll be able to build strength without heavy weights but in fact, the latest research shows that low-intensity resistance training can produce the same results as high-intensity resistance training. In other words, your muscles will respond to Pilates by producing the same gains in muscle strength, size and tone as you would get with other types of resistance training.

However, Pilates doesn't derive its results solely from resistance work. There are a few specific elements that are particular to Pilates. For one, it works in 3D. Each movement is organised with all angles and shapes in mind so that you target your muscles from many different directions. Rather than focus on single-plane movements, Pilates works in a multi-planar fashion.

Additionally, Pilates is dynamic training. While it occasionally demands static holds, the choreography of the system is intended to force the muscles to strengthen while moving.

Finally, Pilates focuses on core training, which you'll be learning all about on the next page. By training your core so that it can support the rest of your body effectively, you'll not only exercise more safely, but you'll be able to exercise more intensely than before.

What's your baseline?

Test your strength with the following Pilates moves. In the Beginner programme some of the exercises you'll meet are the Roll-Back (see p.72), the Swan Prep (see p.83) and the Wall: Chair (see p.98).

• Perform each of these exercises as a baseline assessment on your first day.

• Using a scale of 1 to 10, with 1 being no effort at all and 10 being extremely challenging, rate and note down each exercise according to your experience.

• Repeat the exercises in six weeks and rate them again. Compare your new ratings with the old ones.

UNIFORM DEVELOPMENT
A balanced body has its strength well distributed. Pilates allows uniform development of the body, as Joe Pilates recommended.

Smaller muscle groups like the abdominal obliques and the serratus anterior never get a free ride with Pilates. Everything works all the time.

Postural muscles such as the erector spinae are addressed in Pilates. These muscles work all day long, so they also need strengthening.

Larger muscle groups such as the quadriceps are developed but not over-developed with regular Pilates practice.

Stability

Stability is defined as a resistance to change. As our bodies endure the effects of daily work, repetitive motions and the natural process of ageing, we become less stable and more prone to negative changes. It's these negative changes that we seek to avoid when training with the Pilates method.

The human body is not, by design, a stable structure. The spine is a poor support system for two-legged creatures. Our skulls are too heavy for our bodies and many of our organs are virtually unprotected by any bony structure. However, the joints and complexes within the skeleton have great potential for stability, making the entire structure much more sound.

Pilates professionals often use the example of a chain link to define the effect of one part of the body upon the rest of it. Specifically, a chain is only as strong as its weakest link. Our skeletons have naturally occurring points of strength alternating with points of increased mobility where strength is reduced. Pilates seeks to balance these points by increasing mobility and strength across the skeleton, thereby improving overall structural stability.

Among the advantages you'll gain from improving your stability are the following:

- An improvement in functional fitness – the activities you perform every day.
- Prevention of injury and strain to the spine.
- Improved performance in sports.
- Secondary strength and stability gains in both the hips and the knees.

ALL WORKING TOGETHER
It takes a lot of muscles to be truly stable. The Star exercise demonstrates how the muscles work as a team.

It's all about the core

As it relates to Pilates, stability indicates a stable core, which primarily involves the trunk, or torso, muscles. Your core works all the time whether you're aware of it or not. It helps you lift things up even if they're small. When you unconsciously change your breathing to reach for something or carry something, your core contracts and goes to work. In fact, simply by placing your hand on your abdomen, you can feel this happen. As the load on the muscles increases, the core should contract relative to that workload. If the lower back isn't supported by the core musculature within the body, the back can be strained or injured.

Pilates includes a unique set of core-strengthening exercises and we often employ a system of progressive de-stabilisation to develop the core. This means you may learn an exercise fully supported on your hands and feet and, as you advance, you'll remove one hand, or one leg, or one hand and one leg. By strengthening the body from all angles and working both sides equally, Pilates builds the body from the outside in and the inside out. Your core will stabilise and your physique will be able to resist any negative changes it encounters.

Watchwords!

Watch for these words and phrases as you progress through the exercises in this book. They'll remind you to focus on the stability of your muscles as you exercise.

• Hold strong

• Anchor

• Plant

• Lock down (see p.57)

• Rock solid

The deepest abdominal muscles contract towards the spinal column to prevent the body from losing its balance.

The latissimus dorsi is a key stabilising muscle in this move, stopping the weight of the body from sinking down.

The adductors serve to stabilise both the legs and the pelvis during walking, standing, running and other balancing activities.

The smaller muscles of the arm can't support the weight of the body without the help of the torso,

What's your baseline?

Test your core stabilisation with the following exercise. Grab a timer or stopwatch to begin.

• Assume a plank or push-up position (see p.196, Step 1).

• Keep a straight line from head to toe and hold your abs in strongly.

• Hold this position for as long as possible. Your goal is two minutes.

• Re-test in six weeks. If you achieve two minutes, increase your goal to three minutes. Chart your progress.

Flexibility

In the previous section (see pp.24–5) we discussed the significance of stability. Flexibility is equally important to your overall fitness. Focus on achieving a balance of the two if you want the healthiest possible body.

We define flexibility as "the range of motion in the joint and its surrounding muscles". Tight muscles are limited in their mobility. Muscles that are more flexible can move more efficiently and with a bigger range of motion. For you, this means increased performance with less risk of injury because your limbs will be able to move that much farther before an injury might occur. Bodies come in all shapes and sizes and some people are naturally supple while others aren't. If you're less flexible than you'd like to be, Pilates is ideal.

"If your spine is inflexibly stiff at 30, you are old. If it is completely flexible at 60, you are young."
Joseph Pilates

From origin to insertion

The mechanism of lengthening a muscle simply means that from a muscle's origin (the point at which a muscle's tendons attach to the bone) to its insertion (the far end of the muscle where the same attachment occurs), the distance is increased. This lengthening is most commonly achieved via two distinct methods. The first is known as static stretching. The second is referred to as dynamic stretching and has become the preferred strategy among fitness and medical professionals for becoming more flexible.

During static stretching, you assume your maximum stretch and simply hold it. Beginning at your largest range of motion and sustaining that position has the effect of passively elongating muscle tissue. Holding a leg up in the air to stretch your hamstring or sitting in a straddle stretch (with your legs wide apart on the floor) are examples of static stretching.

During dynamic stretching, you move through a stretching exercise, taking your body into the stretch and back out of it repeatedly. By pairing range-of-motion movements with warm-up-style drills, we simultaneously heat the muscles (which improves the ability of the muscle tissue to extend) as we stretch them. Leg Swings (see pp.143 and 144) and Climb a Tree (see pp.158–9) are examples of dynamic stretching.

In the Pilates method we make the most use of dynamic stretching. Through the repetition of different sequences and the inherently progressive instruction, you'll find your range of motion steadily increasing. If you study

Watchwords!

Watch for these words and phrases as you progress through the exercises in this book. They'll remind you to focus on lengthening and stretching your muscles for increased flexibility.

- Stretch
- Elongate
- Lengthen
- Opposition
- Reach away
- One long line

Pilates in a gym or studio, your teacher may also add a series of static stretches to your routine to promote relaxation and perhaps cool down the body. A regular Pilates practice means you don't need extra stretching.

The benefits of having flexible muscles include:
- Decrease in muscle tension that is often a cause of stress.
- Improvements to misaligned muscles caused by bad postural habits.
- Improved coordination as the nervous system sends messages faster.
- Better circulation.
- Speedier recovery from injury.
- Increased energy from increased blood circulation.

TOUCH THOSE TOES
The Elephant exercise pictured here requires practice if you're inflexible. With consistent effort, your muscles will elongate and become more extensible.

The semitendinosus, semimembranosus and biceps femoris muscles, often referred to jointly as the hamstrings, require persistent stretching to become more flexible.

Lower back pain and tightness are often caused by musculo-ligamentous strain or connective tissue tightness. The quadratus lumborum is one muscle that is frequently responsible for sore backs.

Tight calf muscles – the soleus and gastrocnemius – often protest when they are stretched, which is why you should stretch them regularly.

The muscles of the palms and forearms also contract and become tight. In this position, the flexor digitorum profundis in your forearm gets a chance to lengthen.

What's your baseline?

Test your flexibility with the classic Straight Leg Raise. Perform this sideways in front of a mirror.

- Lie flat on your back with your arms and legs long by your sides.

- Slowly raise one leg as high as you can, keeping it straight. Keep both legs straight. Hold perfectly still.

- Check the mirror and estimate the degree, or ask a friend to take a photo of you. A perfect right angle is 90°.

- Draw a sketch of the angle on a grid so you can see it clearly.

- Re-test yourself in six weeks and compare your results.

Body control

Ever bumped into a piece of furniture that's always been there? Or stumbled off a kerb? When you have developed body control, these instances are far less likely to happen. And when they do happen, you'll be able to respond quicker.

We define body control as a group of abilities that together result in a high degree of movement efficiency and a marked reduction in accident-prone behaviour. Specifically, Pilates improves your timing, balance and motor (or movement) planning so that you waste less time getting from Point A to Point B. You'll also prepare better for accidental outcomes and, most significantly, react faster when the inevitable fumble does occur.

The pieces of the puzzle

Timing isn't something we consciously think about, but bad timing is the primary cause of injuries. When you miss a step on a stairwell or a kerb, bad timing is to blame.

Balance is even more elusive. It isn't the ability to stand on one leg that defines your balance. Rather, it's a balance between the various elements of your body's structure that helps you navigate your day. The ability to move just as far in one direction as the other is a sign of good balance. A body that's restricted in its movement will always struggle to negotiate the course.

Motor planning is the mental and physical process of planning a movement. If you must get to the door, open the door and walk through it, certain processes are involved. These processes go unnoticed by us but they're happening all day long.

Pilates builds control

The Pilates routines in this book begin very simply. You'll repeat certain actions repeatedly within different exercises to develop your timing, balance your body and build muscle memory. As you advance, the material becomes more complex, challenging you in different ways.

An elderly Pilates teacher told me a story once. She was well along in her pregnancy and slipped while stepping into the bath. She automatically went into the Swan exercise (see pp.172–3) – rocking back and forth on her tummy. Is it true? Who knows? But it does illustrate a point. Namely, that Pilates trains your body to handle the unexpected events in life.

"A few well-designed movements, properly performed in a balanced sequence, are worth hours of doing sloppy calisthenics or forced contortion."

Joseph Pilates

Watchwords!

Watch for these words and phrases as you progress through the exercises in this book. They'll remind you to focus on increasing your body control.

- Synchronise
- Simultaneously
- All at once
- Coordinate

What's your baseline?

Test your body control with the following exercise. You'll need a partner to carry this out.

• Find a clutter-free space to stand tall, with a partner nearby. Stand with your legs close together.

• Instruct your partner to lightly push you from several different unexpected directions. The object isn't to make you fall, but to see how fast you can react without falling. Be sure to wait between pushes.

• Note your reaction timing. How much did you stumble? Was one side worse than the other?

• Repeat in six weeks' time and note any changes.

BODY-CONTROL TRAINING
Pilates trains your body control by teaching you to coordinate your mind, body and breath.

BODY

MIND

BREATH

MAKING MUSCLES
Sculpting the Pilates way uses your own body weight and different props, like the weights shown here, to shape and tone your body.

You will see your arm muscles – the biceps, triceps and deltoids – changing shape as you develop your practice.

With Pilates practice your superficial abdominal muscles, such as the rectus abdominis, are toned and tightened together with the deeper muscles like the transversus abdominis.

Attention to alignment can actually reshape your skeleton as your muscles pull your bones into alignment.

Body shape and tone

Muscle tone is defined by the tension in the fibres that make up a muscle while it is at rest. A high degree of muscle tone is visible as well-defined calf muscles or bulging biceps. For many of us, our resting muscle tone is quite poor. In order to improve that tone, there's only one thing you can do and that's exercise.

As you sit, stand or even lie down, your muscles continuously create tension. They receive signals from your brain to fire all day long. The number of individual muscle fibres dictates how much firing must take place.

Body by Pilates

Pilates is ideal for shaping and defining your muscles. Although the mat work utilises only the weight of the body and occasional props for resistance, the system offers full-body conditioning, addressing every part of the body. You may have heard that the abdominals and lower back are the sole focus in Pilates, but a comprehensive Pilates programme will always include upper- and lower-body training.

With regular Pilates practice and a proper diet (see pp.244–9), your body will develop more muscle fibres and decreased body fat. You can expect the fruits of your labour to include visible results such as a flat tummy, strong shoulders, toned back and arms, lean thighs and a high seat.

As well as the actual muscle tone, a Pilates-trained body is distinguished by its graceful carriage and elegant posture. A tight, toned body isn't always the most visible one in the room. It's the body that presents well, with confidence and ease, that really makes heads turn.

Obviously as you develop your flexibility, strength and alignment, your body shape will change. Pilates makes use of negative, or eccentric, loading in order to condition the muscles. This means we contract the muscle in a lengthened position. Technically, this causes micro-tearing in the muscle tissue. The muscle responds by repairing itself, building up more tissue than was there before in a process called hypertrophy. Hypertrophy is how a muscle changes shape (see pp.22–3).

Another means by which Pilates effectively tones the body is by continuous and simultaneous loading. Even while you're performing a Pilates push-up, you'll be asked to contract your glute muscles and thereby train that area as well. This is the Pilates approach. We work everything, all the time.

Watchwords!

Watch for these words and phrases as you progress through the exercises in this book. They'll remind you to focus on the shape and tone of your muscles.

- Resist
- Lift
- Grow
- Firm
- Taut

Endurance

Muscular endurance, or stamina, is a muscle's ability to persist. When you begin your Pilates practice, you'll do just a few repetitions before you feel like stopping and taking a rest. With time, you'll be able to complete the required number of repetitions.

Beginner-level Pilates isn't a steady-state activity like running or cycling. It's more like a circuit-training programme in which you rotate through different activities. But once you become proficient enough and have memorised your programme from start to finish, you'll begin to truly challenge your level of endurance.

Pilates builds muscular endurance both within exercises and also with respect to the entire workout, so you'll need to pay attention to both. Here are a few tips to help you get into a Pilates groove or flow and thereby increase your endurance:

• Cut out extraneous movements – this means no fidgeting!
• Stay focused between movements. Your workout isn't over until the very end.
• Choose a move as your safety net. We all forget what comes next now and then. Pick a move that you like and use it when you slip up or find a move too difficult. Instead, perform your safety-net move. This will buy you time to get back on track.

To hold or not to hold?

Although Pilates workouts don't often include prolonged, static holds, there are occasional moves that help us to improve our endurance. In these instances we continue to find the movements within the sustained hold. Let me give you a perfect example.

In the Wall: Chair exercise (see opposite), you hold a static position. As you hold, tiny movements and adjustments occur as your body tries to cheat. Muscles that have no business working volunteer so that the tired ones can take a break. As your legs become less interested in sustaining the pose, you'll have to shift your focus to other body parts in order to maintain it. You may focus on pressing your skull more firmly into the wall behind you or adjusting your hips so that they stay connected to the wall. Your heels will be trying to lift, so you'll need to force them down. All of this constitutes movement. Perhaps the movements are pretty much imperceptible, but they're still movements. In this way, Pilates is never still or posed and can help increase your endurance.

Watchwords!

Watch for these words and phrases as you progress through the exercises in this book. They'll remind you to focus on increasing your endurance.

• Sustain
• Hover
• Linger
• Suspend

Building endurance

Because Pilates isn't continuous like swimming or running, goal-setting is different. A sample programme to increase your stamina using Pilates might look like this.

Weeks 1–2 Perform 10 exercises with minimum repetitions – keep your form.

Weeks 3–4 Perform 10 exercises with increased repetitions and no break between moves – keep your form.

Weeks 5–6 Perform 10 exercises with maximum reps, no breaks and increased tempo – keep your form.

What's your baseline?

Test your endurance with the Wall: Chair exercise.
Have a stopwatch or a clock with a second hand nearby.

• Stand upright, leaning against a wall with your feet two steps ahead of you.

• Slide down the wall, raising your arms and bending your knees at 90°.

• Maintain the position as long as possible up to two minutes.

• Record your time and check back in six weeks.

Visualising the muscles working can help propel you through sustained exercises. Endurance is also a mental exercise.

Simple body weight is enough to challenge the short but shapely muscles of the shoulders. Here the deltoids do the bulk of the work to suspend the arms.

HOLD JUST A LITTLE LONGER
Building stamina requires commitment, concentration and persistence.

Muscles that span the back and neck work all day to keep you upright. Your paraspinals, or erector spinae, need to build endurance as well.

Endurance exercises often target the large muscle groups such as the quadriceps of the legs, as shown in this move.

Mind over muscle

The phrase "Mind–Body" never seemed to resonate with me. My experience with Pilates seemed so physical, so rigorous and so athletic that this phrase didn't reflect the Pilates workouts I was experiencing. As I began to teach and learned to dissect each move and each sequence, I began to understand the mental connection. To this day, I prefer the phrase "Mind over Muscle" to describe the Pilates process.

From brain to body

It takes an infant almost 30,000 repetitions to perfect a move. What's really happening in that little body is that the nervous system is building a new road. Learning how to move is basically a construction project for the body. Your brain is the foreman supervising the millions of nerves that build the road. Once the road is built, the nerves can travel back and forth along that road to carry out a movement. But until the road is there, a lot of construction must take place.

From body to Pilates body

As you study and practise Pilates, you'll be establishing motor programmes and motor planning. Simply put, this means your ability to plot out and string together movements will become easier. There is a technical process in motor learning that occurs in all human beings who are learning to move. The same process applies to you as you progress from a complete novice to a Pilates pro.

The first stage is called the "cognitive" stage. Here your mind will recognise the images and words in this book and will formulate a plan. Basically, you think about what do to. The second stage of learning Pilates will be your "associative" phase. You'll carry out the moves over and over, all the while refining and perfecting your technique. The final stage is the "automative" stage. When you know your routine so well that you have internalised it, you'll perform each move automatically.

The mental process is translated into a physical one by your central nervous system and specifically by your motor neurons, which carry the electrical impulses that make movement possible. Understood this way, it's easy to see why Joe Pilates was so fond of Friedrich Schiller's remark, "it is the mind itself that shapes the body".

"What is balance of body and mind? It's the conscious control of all muscular movements of the body." Joseph Pilates

Watchwords!

Watch for these words and phrases as you progress through the exercises in this book. They'll remind you to use your mind to move your muscles.

• Visualise

• Imagine

• Picture yourself

• Envisage yourself

What's your baseline?

Test your mind-over-muscle connection with the following exercise, as performed below. Use a mirror to check your results.

• Sit up straight and hug your waist with your arms. Keep your legs long and straight.

• Begin to lower backwards in a reverse sit-up. Don't go too low.

• Close your eyes and try to "see" yourself. Is your stomach out? Shoulders up? Are you crooked?

• Mentally fix everything. Put your body in the perfect shape.

• Open your eyes – did it work? What do you see in the mirror? Note your observations.

• Repeat in six weeks and compare notes.

TALK TO YOURSELF
You must have an internal conversation with your muscles throughout your workout.

Your central nervous system is full of pathways from the brain to every area of the body.

Remember this

Your memory will be key to your Pilates practice. There's no way round it – you simply must memorise your programme. The timed sequences in this book will help you, but I recommend you simply create your own cheat sheet. Take a moment to hand-write your programme. Physically transferring the information from your mind to a piece of paper will help you commit the order of movements to memory. Once you have a memorised list in your head, you no longer need to waste time pausing between moves or fumbling through the book to see what's coming next. You can give your full attention to the quality of your workout, ensuring your rapid progress.

The electrical impulse arrives where the nerve meets the muscle – the neuromuscular junction – and a muscle contraction results.

Stress reduction

Negative stress is toxic. Chronic stress affects your body much as a slow, poisonous leak would. All of your systems are affected. Your digestive system, circulatory, nervous and musculoskeletal systems all suffer. When it comes to exercise as a stress-reduction method, it turns out a little goes a long way.

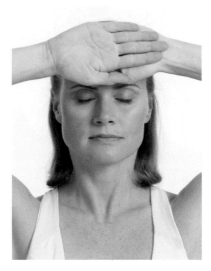

TAKE A MOMENT
Simple warm-up moves can help restore a feeling of wellbeing.

Frequent exercise is one of the best physical stress-reduction strategies available. Even though we know we ought to work out, it can be difficult to imagine how much better we'll feel afterwards. Consider the obvious benefits exercise has on reducing stress:

• Exercise relaxes tense muscles, which contribute to feeling stressful.
• Exercise releases endorphins, which, in turn, improve our mood.
• Exercise helps promote sleep, which dramatically offsets the negative effects of stress.

There's one other interesting benefit that's not often discussed. Exercise seems to give your body a chance to practise dealing with stress. When all of your body's physiological systems are taxed (as they are when you exercise), these systems have to connect and communicate with each other to make your body's responses more efficient and effective. This enhanced information relay is invaluable for your overall wellbeing. It trains your body by means of good stress to handle the effects of bad stress.

Pilates particulars

Is Pilates any better than any other exercise at helping to offset negative stress? I would argue, yes. There are several reasons why I think Pilates stands alone as a training regimen that effectively reduces stress.

FIRST, Pilates promotes breathing that is synchronised with movements. A person with a Pilates-trained body is more likely to stop and take a few breaths during times of stress. This leads to greater mental clarity and a lowered incidence of irrational outbursts.

SECONDLY, Pilates' focus on posture and alignment makes movement feel easier. Poor body mechanics and chronic pain are diminished, which leads to a healthier, easier, physicality.

FINALLY, the body control you develop with Pilates will greatly reduce the day-to-day incidents and accidents that cause us injury and aggravation.

Fuel your workout

Can you completely avoid all negative stress? Probably not. But you can redirect your negative stress to serve you well. Here's a useful tool to turn your bad stress into "eustress", or positive stress. The next time you're hopping mad or feeling aggressive or angry, use that adrenaline to help fuel your workout. Consider it a way of purging the negative waste from your body. Whether you respond better to quick energetic moves or slow steady ones, exercise can help flush out your stress and bring you back into an optimal functional state where you feel and perform your absolute best.

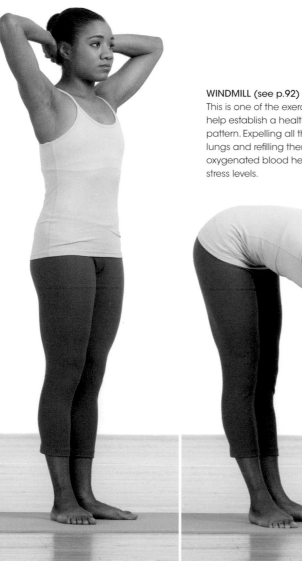

WINDMILL (see p.92)
This is one of the exercises that help establish a healthy breathing pattern. Expelling all the air in the lungs and refilling them with newly oxygenated blood helps to lower stress levels.

Watchwords!

Watch for these words and phrases as you progress through the exercises in this book. They'll remind you to reduce any negative stress as you move.

• Melt

• Relax

• Heavy

• Sink

• Fluidly

• Float

What's your baseline?

Test your stress level with this simple stress-assessment tool:

Rate the following five items on a scale of 1 to 5, with 1 being the worst score (for example, I have headaches all the time, or I have chronic digestive problems) and 5 being the best possible score.

Sleep	1	2	3	4	5
Digestion	1	2	3	4	5
Skin	1	2	3	4	5
Headaches	1	2	3	4	5
Mood swings	1	2	3	4	5

• Tally your results. Anything below 15 means you're under a fair amount of stress.

• Re-test after six weeks of regular practice and note any changes.

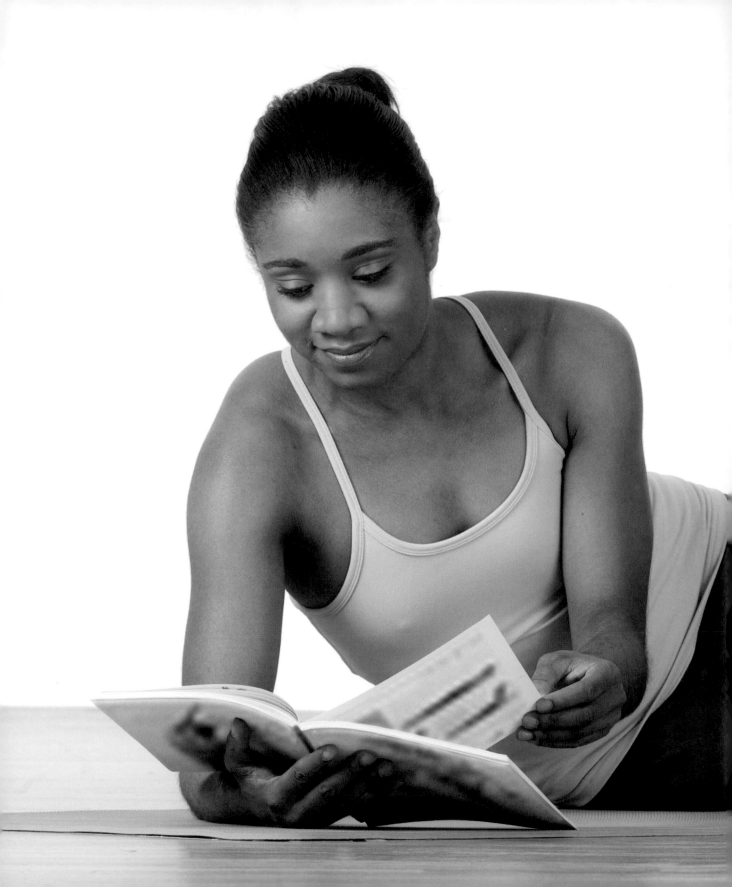

Before
You Begin

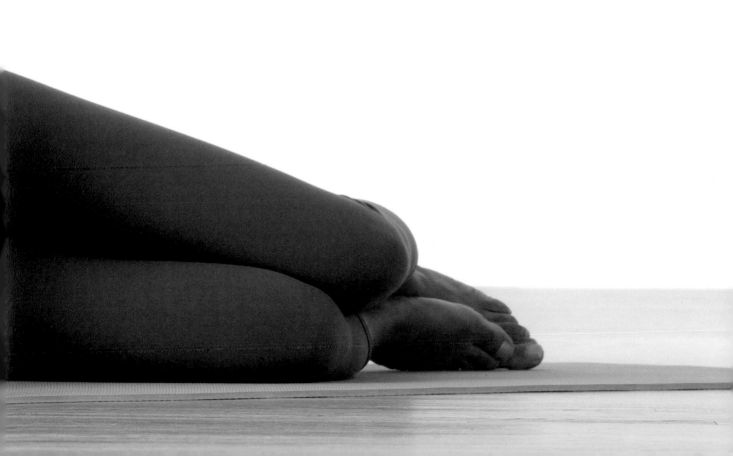

Learning the basics

Having seen what Pilates can do for you, it's time to explore some of the ideology behind Pilates. This chapter is mainly devoted to the six key principles of Pilates. You'll also read some questions and answers about the creation of the programme in this book. And finally, you'll see what tools you'll need to begin your Pilates journey.

Learn now, do later

Before you can practise law, you must study the law. Doctors similarly must learn before doing. Approach Pilates in this way. Study the material, the moves and the history all before you attempt to work out. I recommend you read both of Joe Pilates' original titles, *Your Health* and *Return to Life through Contrology*. By the time you get started, you'll have such a deep understanding of the work, you'll already have begun to transform your body.

Do now, ask later

In the organisation of this book, I was guided by the six principles. Each move you'll learn was crafted according to one of the principles. Moreover,

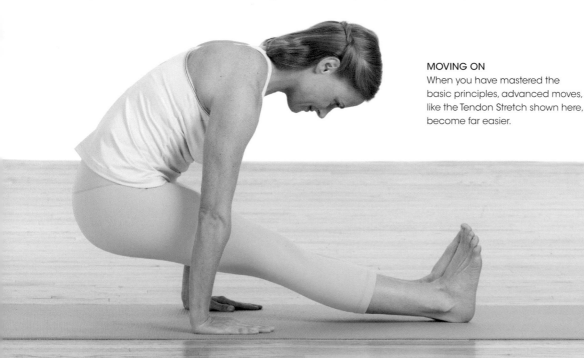

MOVING ON
When you have mastered the basic principles, advanced moves, like the Tendon Stretch shown here, become far easier.

the sequences of exercises were constructed according to these founding principles. Initially, I listed all of the moves in Mr Pilates' original programme (see p.50) and studied the patterns Mr Pilates followed. When it was time to create the full programmes, I continually referred to these principles. But as the book got closer to being done, it became time to ask questions. Many questions arose during the writing of this book and in attempting to answer them I found myself returning to Mr Pilates' writings and his basic principles. As you develop your practice, questions may arise. Seek answers in Mr Pilates' work and in the basic ideas of the system.

What do you want?

One of the questions you must ask yourself is "What do I want from Pilates?" As you read through the section on the six principles, begin to think about what you really want from your Pilates programme. Rather than mindlessly exercising, take the opportunity to map out a mental plan. Your goals are key to your success. Take the time to set a reasonable goal that you'll be able to achieve with consistency. Your goals don't have to be technical or formal. They can be simply laid out. For example:

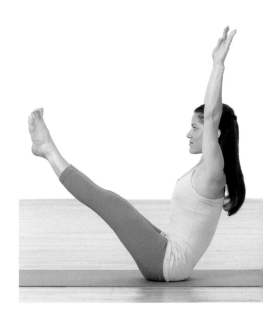

A SYNTHESIS OF ALL THE PRINCIPLES
Exercises like Teaser III, shown here, require you to synthesise all the principles of Pilates.

SAMPLE FLEXIBILITY GOAL
• **TEST** January 1: Straight Leg Raise – leg only able to raise to a diagonal and not straight.
• **SET GOAL** March 1: Be able to straighten leg more and higher. Aim for leg to be fully straight and directly to the ceiling.
• **RE-TEST** March 1: So close! Fully straight but not quite there yet.

What do you need?

All goals need a plan of execution and the necessary tools. You'll find all the equipment you'll need is neatly laid out in this section (see pp.52–3). There's no need to over-prepare. Get only what you need. Pilates is very low-tech.

The heart of Pilates

As you embark upon your Pilates life, be certain to re-read these pages periodically. When you hit a plateau or decide to try a new workout or just don't feel motivated, read about the six principles once more. Get back to the heart of Pilates with these concepts and bring them back into your workout. I'm certain that you can find inspiration within the original principles and ideals of the Pilates work. The fun will be to make them your own.

The six Pilates principles

Joe Pilates was committed to developing a system that addressed all aspects of wellness. In his books, he outlined his six principles. These were meant to serve as a theoretical basis for his work. They don't teach us how to sit up or how to do push-ups, but rather how to approach the Pilates body of work.

It's impossible to know exactly what Mr Pilates had in mind when he created his list of six principles, or even if he might have adjusted them given more time. Over the years, many of his disciples and students have added to the list so that teacher-training programmes now vary in what they define as the guiding principles of Pilates.

Of course, there are many concepts that ultimately influence a practitioner's approach to the Pilates method, but in order to experience Pilates the way Joe intended us to, it's always best practice to begin at the beginning. To study Pilates properly you must begin with the six principles.

The following pages explore the ideas behind each of the six principles. My interpretations accompany each principle. I invite you to consider alternative interpretations as your execution of Pilates grows and improves.

Control

Control is the mother ship of all the Pilates principles and is the one principle for which Pilates named his fitness methodology. "Contrology" was the moniker Pilates chose as the official label of his system, but during his lifetime the system was also known as the "Universal Method". It wasn't until many years later that it came to be known simply as Pilates. But to return to our first principle. Control what?, you may wonder. And the answer is a resounding "everything". If you learn only one principle, it must be the principle of Control.

Learning to control your movements is the foundation of Pilates. Don't assume this means your movements become slow and stuck. Quite the opposite, in fact. Your mastery of the Control principle dictates that you must be able to move at a rapid pace without ever losing control. Your mind, your muscles and your ability are all under your control. Think for a moment about how much control you must utilise simply to put an exercise plan into action. Deciding to become fit, showing up every day and performing to your absolute best all demonstrate enormous control. Pilates requires you to exercise that control and, more importantly, it helps you to develop it.

Alycea's Pilates rule book

Memorising six words won't be as effective as understanding the six ideas that govern your Pilates practice. These short phrases will help you remember the six principles and the ideas behind them.

1 Take **control**.

2 Concentration is the key.

3 Centre the mind in/move from the centre out.

4 "Almost" doesn't count. Be **precise**.

5 Breath is life.

6 Ebb and **flow**.

Concentration

Concentration is often referred to using that fitness-industry buzzword "mindfulness". Pilates was early in adopting mindfulness as a basis of his work. He always stated that one of the primary benefits of his method was "complete coordination of body, mind and spirit". This is impressive for an exercise culture that was still on the periphery of the mind–body fitness we know today.

Nowadays, fitness professionals understand that to accomplish the best results, complete concentration is key. All the more so with Pilates. The Pilates method is complex. And while it can be practised at any level from remedial through super-advanced, your practice will only be as effective as your concentration. Work out while you're distracted and you may get your heart rate up, but work out with total concentration and you'll work out harder and longer and you'll get results faster.

Your concentration can waiver, so don't overwhelm yourself by trying to focus on every part of your body all at once. Instead, while you exercise, focus on one part of your body. Over time, your focus will strengthen and you'll find you can concentrate on everything at once.

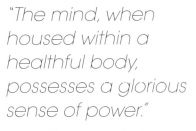

"The mind, when housed within a healthful body, possesses a glorious sense of power."

Joseph Pilates, in a letter to a client, 1939

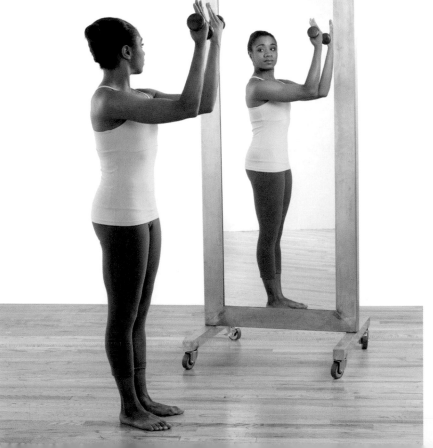

HOW DO I LOOK?
Watching yourself in front of a mirror while you work out can help to focus your mind on your body.

Centring

Having dictated that we should use total control and also be completely mindful in our practice, Mr Pilates designated Centring as his third principle. Marrying movement from your physical centre with the action of centring your mind sets the stage for powerful exercise. One of Joe Pilates' disciples used to say that each and every move we perform in Pilates is movement "flowing out from a strong centre".

Centring your mind is key to the practice of Pilates. Try to work out in a distraction-free environment. If you find your focus drifting away, return to the beginning of the exercise and start again.

Your physical "centre" for the purpose of Pilates extends from your upper abdominals down to your upper thighs. It includes your pelvic-floor muscles and gluteals. In Pilates, this area is also known as the "powerhouse" (see p.61).

To promote your use of centring during your practice, I recommend two strategies. First, begin each and every movement by initiating from your centre. This means some activity should occur in your midsection. Your abs may contract, firm, or tighten or you may just become suddenly aware of that part of your body.

Second, be sure to end each and every movement by returning your focus to your centre. For many of us, the middle of the exercise is a time when details are lost and attention waivers. Before you finish any exercise, pause. Re-connect to the centre of your body and, only then, move on to the next movement.

Centring is fundamental to your practice and no matter how experienced you become, you'll always be able to take this principle one step further.

PULL IN AND UP
Without a focus on the centre of the body, exercises like this one are impossible to achieve.

Precision

Mr Pilates wrote that his method should be executed in the prescribed order, with the prescribed breathing protocol and for the prescribed number of repetitions. In his studio, these rules were routinely adjusted, but from his writings, it's clear that he intended his system to be predictable and easily duplicated for the home user. For your own practice, keep a precise list of exercises in an exact order and with a certain number of repetitions each.

Precision doesn't come easy. I'm a stickler for preparation. "Be prepared or be prepared to fail" is an appropriate sentiment when you're looking to accomplish specific, measurable goals. Approach Pilates as both a study and a discipline. If you work sloppily without attention to detail or precision, you'll certainly fail at your exercise objectives. But with that attention, you can achieve your desired results. To foster precision in your practice, you must have as much information as possible. Make absolutely sure you know all the rules, steps and goals for each move before you execute it. And of course, practice makes perfect.

There are many areas of your practice where you can focus on precision. Within each exercise, try to give each movement equal significance. I repeatedly emphasise to my students that no part of any exercise is more important than any other part. Attack each move from this perspective.

The time taken between exercises is also an opportunity to practise precision. Transitioning between each exercise should be done with a minimum of movement to promote maximum efficiency. Use the quickest means to get where you need to go next.

I'm certain that Mr Pilates was never satisfied that his work was enough and that he always felt there was more he could do with his system. Striving for precision is part of the Pilates game plan. Continue to push yourself forward, one principle and one step at a time.

SETUP IS KEY
To get the most out of each exercise, each part of the movement should be precisely executed.

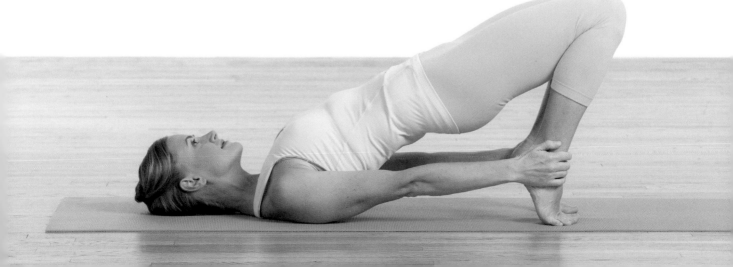

Breath

Volumes can be written about Mr Pilates' approach to breathing. He wrote about it profusely in his books and even created a device specifically to address breathing capacity. He called this apparatus the Breath-a-Cizer (see photograph below). It consists of a little wheel mounted on a handle, with a holder for a drinking straw. Students blow through the straw and see how long they can keep the wheel turning with one single exhalation. With regular Pilates practice, students can improve their breathing tremendously. The Breath-a-Cizer is a forerunner of the peak-flow meter that doctors use nowadays to test lung function.

Pilates was right to address breathing as fundamental. Proper oxygen uptake is key to optimal function. By focusing on the breath as part of the choreography of his exercise system, he was essentially instructing us to send oxygen to the working muscles. He likened inhaling to the inflating of a balloon and exhaling to the wringing out of a towel. He suggested that we breathe as follows:

- **INHALE FROM THE TOP** down to the base of the lungs.
- **EXHALE FROM THE BASE** up and out through the top.

There are other schools of thought on the Pilates breathing technique, most developed after Mr Pilates' time. Many, if not most, instructors now teach what's known as lateral breathing. In lateral breathing you take in air and expand your rib cage to accommodate your expanding lungs. Rather than expand the abdominal wall, the breather focuses on sending air into the back and sides of the body in order to keep the centre strong and firm.

You may experience other breathing methods as you explore Pilates classes and lessons. Whichever alternative techniques you add to your breathing repertoire later, always return to the basics.

PRACTISE AT HOME
You don't need a Breath-a-Cizer (left) to increase your breath capacity. Use your imagination and concentration to help you practise slow, controlled inhalations and exhalations.

Flow

If you've ever gone for a long bike ride or a jog through the park, you've probably experienced how good it feels to get into a rhythm or flow. The same is true for sports, dance or martial arts and, of course, for Pilates. You establish your flow, then keep it up. In Pilates we strive to perform our workouts at a steady pace that mimics the rhythm of our heart.

Joe Pilates didn't intend his method to be performed staccato or in sections. Instead, he dictated that one exercise should move neatly into the next, with no wasted movements. Watching the old films and seeing Mr Pilates' official mounting and dismounting postures for many of his machine-based moves, you can clearly see this idea in action.

Work hard to join your Pilates exercises together, creating one long routine without any real rests between movements. From setting up your mat to wiping your brow after your workout, all your moves should be connected. In this way, you'll create a workout that truly flows, keeping your heart rate elevated and increasing your endurance as added benefits.

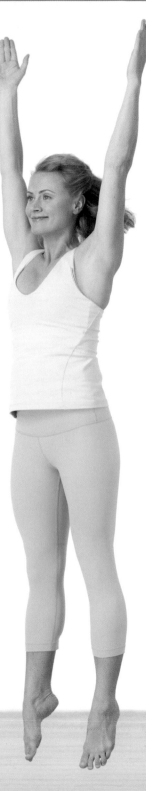

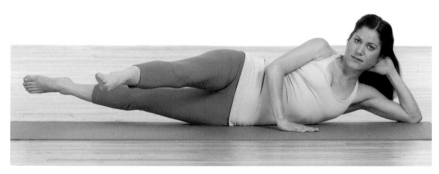

BACK AND FORTH
Exercises like the Side Kicks: Scissors (see p.131) help you connect movements together.

UP AND DOWN
Jumping is a natural way to experience flowing movement.

Six Pilates principles in one exercise

The beauty of Pilates is that it can be adjusted, adapted and modified to target any weakness or body part that we deem necessary. I often say I can make a whole workout for your little finger if need to. To see how simple it is to shift gears from one principle to another, take a look at one exercise approached in several different ways. To the objective eye, there may be no difference. But to the practitioner, there's a tremendous difference in the way he or she experiences these moves.

I routinely tell my students that Pilates "works as hard as you do". Layering in these six Pilates principles will absolutely make your workout harder.

1 Control

To focus on the first principle – Control – the objective is to establish a strong and solid position. From the beginning through to the end, there should be no extraneous movements or uncertain motions. The entire exercise should look like a well-rehearsed performance.

2 Concentration

Once the focus changes to Concentration, the student must shift into mental mode. I usually recommend you "speak to yourself". Spell out the move and the steps in your mind. Become your own teacher, taking yourself through one move at a time. Correct what you see and what you know are your weak spots. Don't let your mind wander.

3 Centring

To emphasise the third principle of Centring, visualisation is key. Now you can merge the mental and the physical, bringing all the attention towards the middle of your body. Imagine activating your centre before you even assume your first position. And as the movement concludes, the centre of your body should be the strongest part of your anatomy.

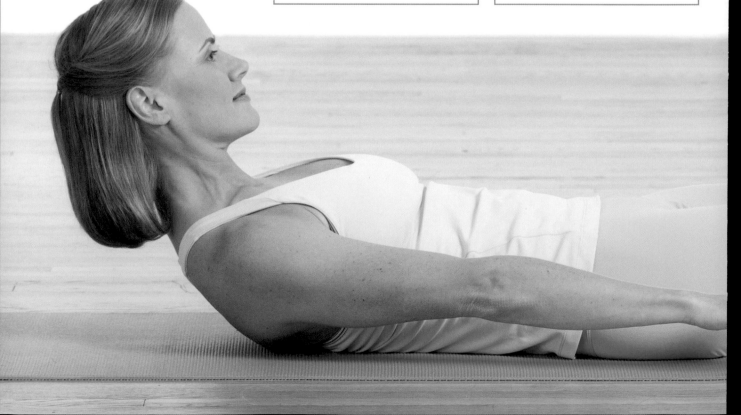

When you start practising Pilates, it's important to experiment with your focus. The list of exercises you perform will remain constant depending upon which programme you choose. But by rotating your focus through the six principles, you'll find new ways to improve your form and intensify your workout. To help you memorise the principles, practise them in the order below. You don't have to focus on every principle each time you practise a move, but on days that you rehearse them all, perform them in the order laid out below.

Let's dissect a classic Pilates move – The Hundred – often the first to be performed in a programme.

4 Precision

The Pilates practitioner demonstrates Precision in very much the same way as a gymnast would – performing a strong setup leading into a perfect execution and a solid ending. Precision is evident in the student's form, timing and tempo. In this example of The Hundred, the height and rotation of the legs are essential to help evaluate the student's precision.

5 Breath

The fifth principle of Pilates is demonstrated quite nicely in The Hundred. In what is essentially a breathing exercise, the student must focus on the tempo and flow of the breath in order to execute the move properly. To focus on Breath fully and completely, you must also pay attention to the quality and efficiency of the breath.

6 Flow

A more experienced student will routinely make use of the Flow principle. But beginners take heed. It will serve you well to practise connecting your moves to your breath. You should also become adept at stringing together your setup, execution and conclusion from the beginning of your practice. Within each individual exercise, keep a smooth, even quality.

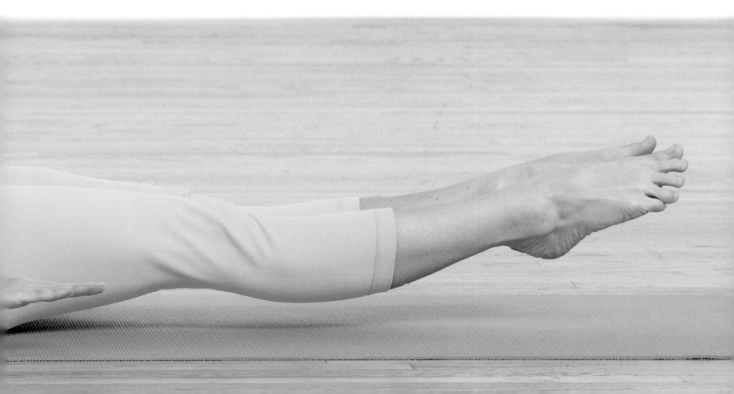

Pilates Qs and As

The exercise routines you are about to embark upon are a completely original Pilates sequencing. They are a set of unique programmes that I have organised according to my teaching experience over the last two decades.

Mr Pilates' original exercises

You'll find most of these exercises in this book.

1 The Hundred
2 The Roll-Up
3 The Roll-Over with Legs Spread
4 The One-Leg Circle
5 Rolling Back
6 The One-Leg Stretch
7 The Double-Leg Stretch
8 The Spine Stretch
9 Rocker with Open Legs
10 The Corkscrew
11 The Saw
12 The Swan-Dive
13 The One-Leg Kick
14 The Double Kick
15 The Neck Pull
16 The Scissors
17 The Bicycle
18 The Shoulder Bridge
19 The Spine Twist
20 The Jackknife
21 The Side Kick
22 The Teaser
23 The Hip Twist
24 Swimming
25 The Leg-Pull – Front
26 The Leg-Pull
27 The Side Kick – Kneeling
28 The Side Bend
29 The Boomerang
30 The Seal
31 The Crab
32 The Rocking
33 The Control Balance
34 The Push-Up

I'm a true advocate of the pure, classical Pilates method, or what I call "real Pilates", as the launchpad for all Pilates training. For that reason, almost all of Mr Pilates' original 34 exercises (see box, left) are included in this book's programme. Where I've omitted some, it was simply to substitute an exercise borrowed from the archival material or from the syllabus for using Pilates equipment. No two Pilates lessons are alike. Each session brings a new cue, a new emphasis or some nuance to your workout. I've created these workouts for you to experience the broadest possible range. You'll find that adjustments to timing, repetitions and positions have been made in an effort to leave no stone unturned.

Here are some of the questions that arose during the writing of this book. They were posed by students and teachers alike. I hope my answers both satisfy and inspire you.

Q *These moves are different from those in other Pilates books I've seen. Are they the original Pilates moves?*
A Yes they are. I've made small adjustments in position, timing, setup and sequence, but the moves are those of Joe Pilates – not mine. Think of me as the delivery vehicle. Pilates is a tremendous system and can't be contained in the pages of one book. Here you'll experience a variety of moves showing many different aspects of the real Pilates method.

Q *I thought Pilates was done lying on your back. There seem to be a lot of other positions in this book and a lot of standing moves. Are those real Pilates exercises?*
A They certainly are! There's a huge library of Pilates moves done upright and they are very important exercises. The bulk of your waking hours is spent upright. You ought to exercise in order to address that reality. That's why I always include upright exercises in your programme.

Q *Is there a reason you chose to re-arrange certain movements? For example, some moves seem to start at the end and work their way backwards, rather than the other way round?*

A In my experience of teaching group fitness for almost 20 years, I've observed that most people are able to accomplish certain moves if they're performed from an easier starting point. When you begin any new exercise programme, confidence is key to improving. Reversing certain exercises makes this easier to accomplish.

Q *How did you decide which exercises were to be included in your Beginner, Intermediate and Advanced programmes?*
A For this book, I selected the simplest mechanical movements as the Beginner moves. That doesn't mean that they are the easiest to accomplish. But they are the simplest to instruct and execute when you break down the movement into its component parts. A simple squat or bicep curl is one single movement and most people can perform it even though they may find it difficult. Movements that encompass choreography and extra components are the ones that I have slotted into the Intermediate and Advanced programmes.

Q *I thought the Pilates order was always the same? How did you avoid giving the same programme with the same exercises for the different levels?*
A If you're practising from a list, the order will always be the same. But step into a class anywhere in the world and there's tremendous variation from class to class. The truth is, there are so many exercises to choose from that it's never necessary to repeat the same exact moves.

Q *How do I get from one move to the next? Are there specific choreographed transitions?*
A There are! But they're not included in the step-by-step instructions in this book as we would need many more pages to cover every detail. However, they are included in the Sequences (see pp.104–9, 146–51 and 208–13), which show you how to divide up your workout into 15-, 30-, or 45-minute segments. The most important thing to know about transitioning between exercises is that it should be done as quickly and efficiently as possible.

Q *What determines how many repetitions I should perform?*
A Listen to your body. If I give a range such as 6 to10 reps, do as many as possible in perfect form. Once you start to lose the details, it's time to move on.

Q *Is there a formula for ending each routine?*
A In my personal training, I insist that all students end their routines with a standing move or series of standing moves. This is to bring all the great Pilates work you've done into an upright position and prepare you for your day.

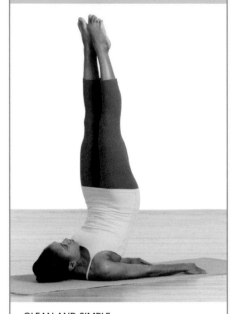

The right clothing

CLEAN AND SIMPLE
Keep your workout clothes form-fitting and simple so as not to distract from your routine. Fitness wear should assist you – not get in the way.

Clothing and equipment

To begin your study and practice of Pilates, there are a few things you will need. Pilates done in the home is remarkably low-tech. But a few tools will help you get the most out of your workout.

First, you'll need a surface to lie on. Pilates mats should be slightly thicker than yoga mats so that your spine is padded. A gymnastics mat will work just fine. If you prefer the thinner, space-saving option of a yoga-style mat, look for one at least ½ centimetre (¼ inch) thick. Don't want to pay out for a mat? You don't really have to. A carpeted floor with some blankets or rolled-up towels will suffice at a pinch.

I've included a few props in this book that you can purchase at a sporting goods shop or on the internet. Small hand weights or dumbbells of 1–2.5kg (2–5lb) are ideal. Exercise bands which are elastic and lightweight are also included in this programme. Make sure to get bands rather than tubing, which functions very differently. You can also use a weighted bar or short pole. If neither of those is available, you may substitute a medium-size playground ball. Finally, I recommend that you work out in front of a mirror whenever possible.

What to wear

ON TOP I recommend all Pilates students wear simple, form-fitting tops. Avoid tops that have jewels or decorative stones. Excess ruching, pleats, ribbons or raised stitching will become uncomfortable within minutes of starting your workout. Be especially aware of the back of the garment, where designers often get creative and place some decorative detail that makes rolling or lying flat simply impossible.

ON THE BOTTOM For your lower half, you have lots of options. Shorts, leggings, or workout trousers are all good choices. Look for comfortable fabric with flat seams and minimal design work. Shorts should hug the body as you will have your legs overhead during the programmes in this book.

GET YOUR GEAR
Pilates props are abundant. These
will enhance your Pilates practice.

A Pilates mat should
be slightly thicker
than a yoga mat

A weighted bar can
be used instead of
an exercise band

Hand weights between
1 and 2.5kg (2 and 5lb)
are ideal

Exercise bands
come in different
resistances
– choose a
medium weight

Grips on your
socks can help
in some upright
exercises

Some socks
separate each toe
for better foot
articulation

Similarly, workout trousers that open too wide at the bottom or fit too loosely
can flop around your legs as you work out, causing a distraction.

ON THE FEET Traditionally, Pilates has been done barefoot. As studios began
to serve the masses, many began to require people to wear socks. For your
home practice, you can choose to go bare or cover up your feet. If you
prefer socks, you can choose between plain socks or sticky socks that grip
the floor. There are even toe socks that separate each individual toe.

ELSEWHERE Be sure to strip off any jewellery, watches or glasses before you
begin. Long hair should be pulled back neatly. It's best if you work out in a
ventilated space and, of course, always keep some water handy.

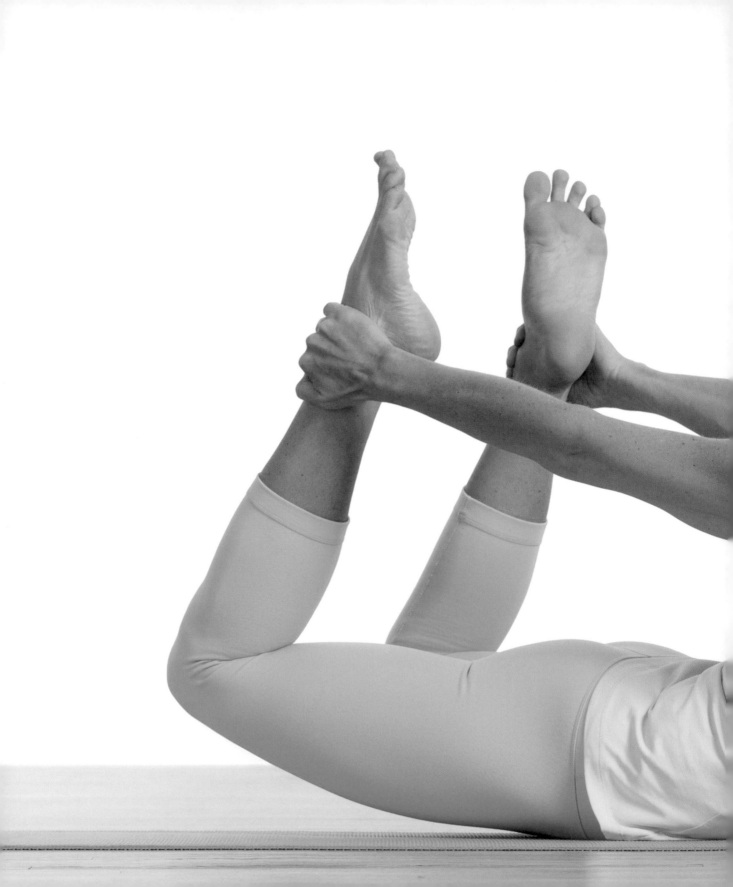

The Exercises

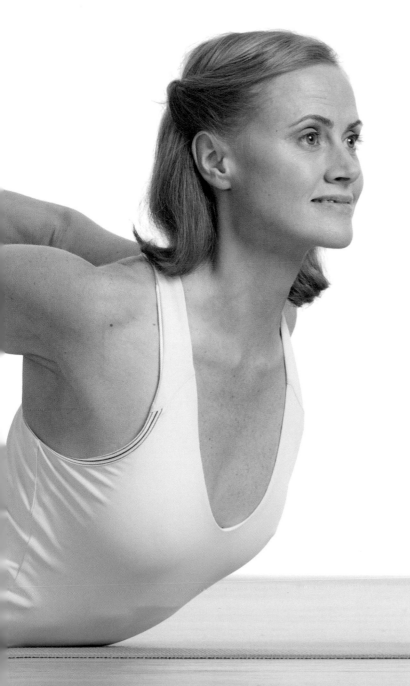

How this book works

In this book you will find a short Warm-Up (see pp.60–65) that is intended to introduce you to the key movement concepts in Pilates. Complete Beginner, Intermediate and Advanced-level programmes follow the Warm-Up. After each of these programmes you will find timed routines for performing a 15-minute, 30-minute or full 45-minute workout, as your schedule permits. Learn the Warm-Up and practise it before your workout until you have integrated it into your Pilates practice.

The exercises

Each exercise has been laid out to give you all the information you could possibly need. Below the exercise name you'll see a "Focus On" line, which provides you with a keyword relating to one of the six Pilates principles (see pp.42–9). Bear this keyword in mind as you practise. It will give you a specific focus for each exercise.

Many exercises include an inset photo labelled Common Faults. Here you will see incorrect form and common mistakes that new students make. In some instances, an exercise includes a modification to make a move harder (Ready for a challenge?) or simpler (Too hard? Try this).

Breathing instructions have been woven into the step-by-step instructions so that you'll know when and where to emphasise the breathing.

HOW MANY AND HOW FAST?

Each exercise also includes a box that tells you how many repetitions you should be performing as well as how fast or slow to go. Under the "How many do I do?" heading, you'll find a few variations. If you're perfoming a move that doesn't involve switching sides, you'll be instructed to perform a certain number of reps, or repetitions.

For exercises where you switch sides, you'll be instructed to perform sets. A set consists of one rep to the right and one to the left. Therefore 5 sets would equal 10 reps. Be sure to note how many reps or sets are assigned to a given exercise.

Periodically you'll see instructions to alternate directions. And occasionally, you'll have to perform all your repetitions to one side before beginning again on the other side.

Even with all of the guidance and information in this book, Pilates can't be learned overnight. Take your time, enjoy the journey, and have fun!

A tempo to suit you

Tempo varies from exercise to exercise. To keep you working at a proper pace, here is a simple formula.

Resting breathing frequency, or the number of breaths you take per minute, falls somewhere between 12 and 20 breaths. When an exercise is labelled SLOW, your breathing frequency should be between 20 and 25 breaths per minute. For MODERATE exercises, 25 to 30 and for FAST, 30 to 35 breaths per minute.

For an additional gauge to how hard you should be working, follow the Maximum Speed column below. For each tempo, you should be working at a percentage of your personal maximum. So SLOW will coordinate with 10% to 35% of your own maximum speed.

Tempo	Breathing frequency	Maximum speed
SLOW	20–25	10–35%
MODERATE	25–30	35–60%
RAPID	30–35	60–80%

AT-A-GLANCE
Each exercise is chock-full of details that provide you with all the information you need.

Level Note the colour tab that identifies the level of difficulty of the exercise.

Intro Find out a little about the exercise and pick up extra tips with the Intro material.

How many do I do? and **Tempo** Find out exactly how much to do and how fast to go.

Focus on This indicates the Pilates principle to focus on in each exercise.

Step-by-step photos All the steps are clearly labelled in numerical order to guide you through the movement.

Modification Learn how to adjust to make the move easier or harder.

Annotations These accompany each photo to provide additional details or simply to emphasise an action.

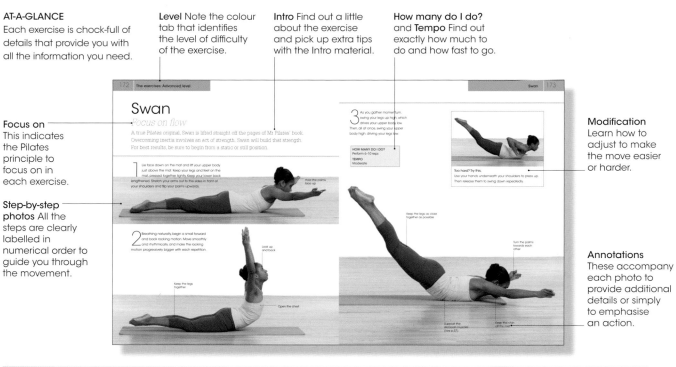

Glossary

NOUN	MIGHT ALSO SAY	WHAT IT MEANS
Abs	Midsection; abdominals; waistline	The muscles in the front of your torso that span from your ribs down to your pelvis
Box	Frame; keep your box square; work within your frame	The action of keeping your torso squarely aligned so that your shoulders and hips create a symmetrical square-like shape
Isometric	–	Exercise that doesn't involve movement
Midline	Centre line	An imaginary line down the middle of your body
Pilates stance	Make a small "V"; rotate into a letter "V"	Rotate your legs and feet into a small "V"
Powerhouse	Core; centre	The power centre of your body, including your abs, buttocks and inner thighs
Resistance	Opposition	Working your muscles against a force
Tail	Buttocks; seat	The bottom you sit on!

VERB	MIGHT ALSO SAY	WHAT IT MEANS
Anchor	Lock down; hold strong; support; strong posture	The action of tightening your muscles so they hold their position as well as holding your body in position
Articulate	Roll through; one vertebra at a time	The movement of each bone or part of the body in sequence, as when you roll through the spine
Curl	Crunch; round	The act of rounding your spine to pull the abdominals inwards
Fire up	Contract; activate	The action of tensing or hardening a muscle
Scoop	Hollow; navel to spine; navel towards spine; cinch the waist; pull the abs in and up	The action of pulling the abdominals in and up at the same time so that the waist narrows

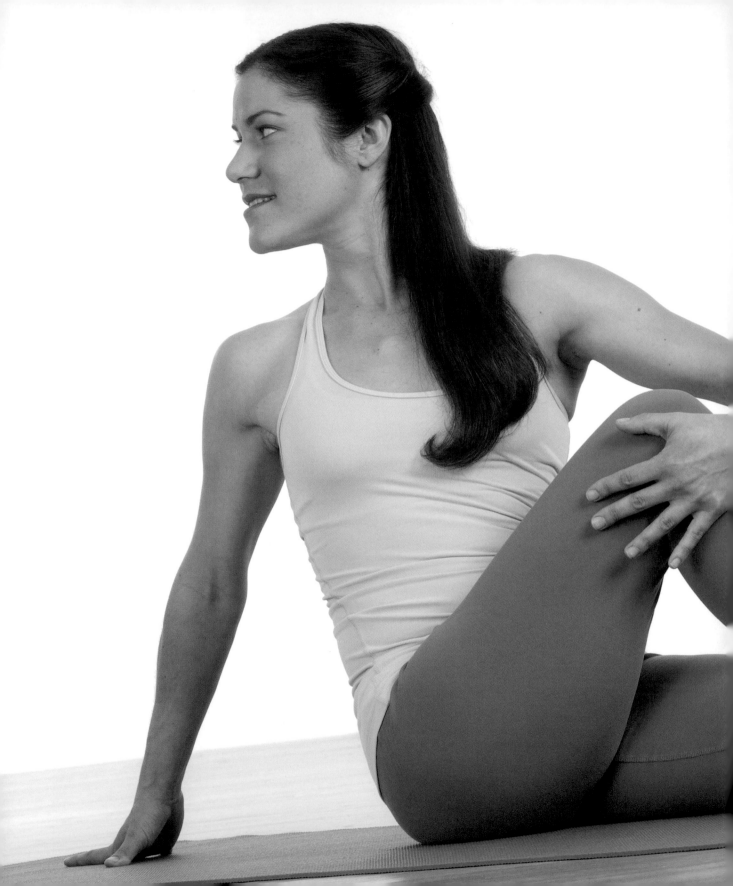

Warm-Up

Warming up your body can do more than just generate heat. A good Pilates warm-up also sets you up for your workout by establishing the anatomical rules that your body will follow throughout the rest of your exercise.

Standing Rotation
Focus on Pilates stance

You will do many of your Pilates exercises with your heels together and your toes apart. This is what we call "Pilates stance". It involves working the muscles of your backside, also known as your gluteal muscles.

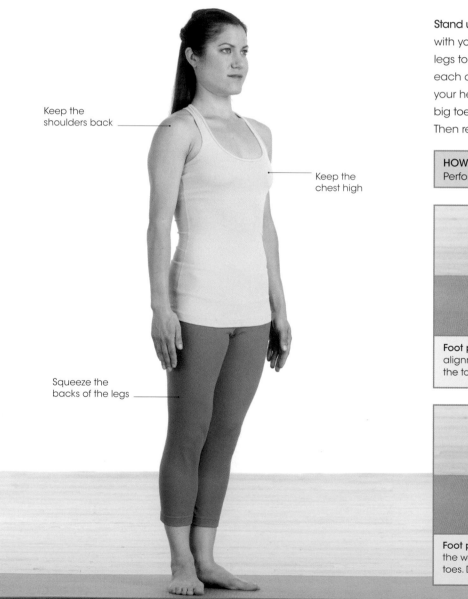

Keep the
shoulders back

Keep the
chest high

Squeeze the
backs of the legs

Stand upright in your best posture (see pp.20–21) with your arms down by your sides. Bring your legs together and take your feet parallel to each other (position A). Rock back slightly on your heels and tense your glutes so that your big toes separate 5–7.5cm (2–3in) (position B). Then release your glutes and close your feet.

HOW MANY DO I DO?
Perform 5 reps

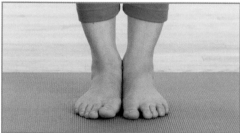

Foot position A Your feet must begin in good alignment. Be sure that the heels are level and the toes are together.

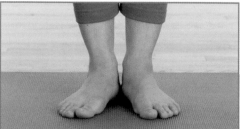

Foot position B As you open your feet, keep the weight of your body equally over all ten toes. Don't roll out or in.

Activation
Focus on the powerhouse

Your powerhouse consists of your abdominals, your gluteals and your pelvic-floor muscles – in other words, your "core". Never tuck, crunch or round your spine to activate your core. As you practise, imagine you are "scooping up your abs".

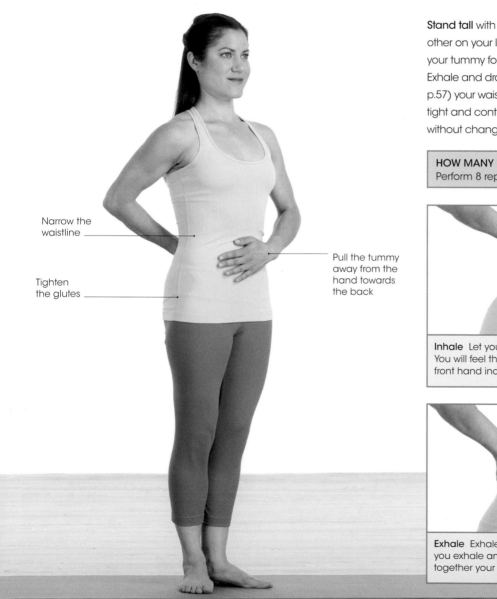

Narrow the waistline

Tighten the glutes

Pull the tummy away from the hand towards the back

Stand tall with one hand on your abs and the other on your lower back. Inhale and release your tummy forward into your hand (below, top). Exhale and draw your abs in, cinching (see p.57) your waist (below, bottom). Keep your glutes tight and contract your pelvic-floor muscles without changing the position of your spine.

HOW MANY DO I DO?
Perform 8 reps

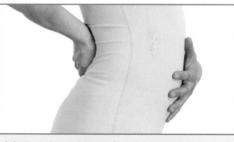

Inhale Let your tummy fill with air as you inhale. You will feel the distance from back hand to front hand increase.

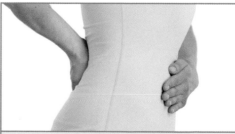

Exhale Exhale to empty the air. The more you exhale and contract the waist, the closer together your two hands will come.

Four Corners
Focus on the box or frame

Alignment is key to the practice of Pilates. Your upper body creates a "box" or "frame", from shoulder to shoulder and hip to hip. The box is a constant reference to keep you square and safe as you practise.

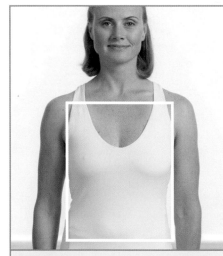

The box Your torso makes a natural frame to keep you in good alignment. Use these 4 corners to check your form.

Come onto all fours on your mat. Place your hands directly under your shoulders and your knees directly under your hips. Keep your weight equally balanced on each limb. Visualise your hands and knees connected by 4 lines that create a box. Take 5 breaths, alternately lifting your abdominals and releasing them with each exhale.

HOW MANY DO I DO?
Perform 5 reps

Maintain a long, straight neck

Keep the legs in a straight line under the hips

Lift the abs

Keep the arms in a straight line under the shoulders

Sit and "C"

Focus on the C-curve

By now you should be able to scoop up your abdominals without changing the position of your spine. The next step is skeletal mobility. Many Pilates exercises require you to make a C-curve with your spine by curving each vertebra, so practise this move a lot.

Sit with your knees bent and your legs almost hip-width apart. Hold behind your knees and round your back forward over your legs to make a "C" shape. Begin inhaling as though you could fill up your lower back with air. With each exhale, scoop your abs up high and round forward more to increase the curve in your spine. Stretch the sides of your waist up to accentuate the "C" shape even more.

HOW MANY DO I DO?
Perform 5 reps

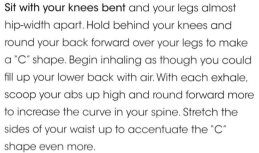

Hang the head

Hold behind the knees

Pull the waist back

Neck Presses

Focus on neck alignment

Neck pain while doing abdominal exercises is very common and deeply frustrating. Learn to tackle those muscles at the outset when you start to learn Pilates. By using simple isometric moves (see p.57), your neck should remain strong and aligned.

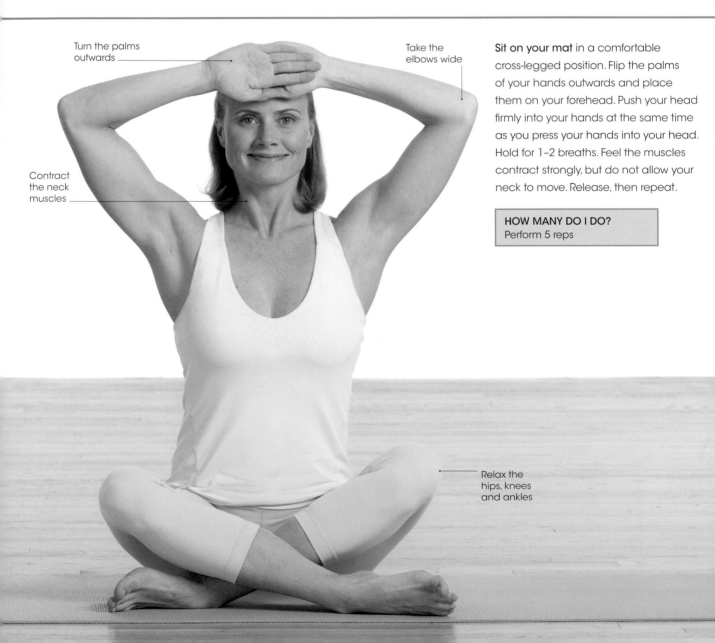

Turn the palms outwards

Take the elbows wide

Contract the neck muscles

Relax the hips, knees and ankles

Sit on your mat in a comfortable cross-legged position. Flip the palms of your hands outwards and place them on your forehead. Push your head firmly into your hands at the same time as you press your hands into your head. Hold for 1–2 breaths. Feel the muscles contract strongly, but do not allow your neck to move. Release, then repeat.

HOW MANY DO I DO?
Perform 5 reps

Pelvic Curl

Focus on spinal articulation

Phrases like "articulate through the spine" and "one vertebra at a time" are a mainstay of the Pilates method. For tight lower backs, Pilates can be truly medicinal. Begin practising this articulation with this simple movement.

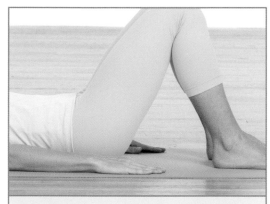

Starting position As you start, be sure to leave your hips and bottom heavy on the mat. There should be no tension in your gluteals before you begin.

Lie on your back with your knees bent up and your legs comfortably apart. Keeping your head and arms down, lengthen your lower back as though you were pulling the vertebrae of your lower back apart. Tilt your hips up, scoop your abs deeply and curl your pelvis up 10–15cm (4–6in) off the mat. Inhale to lower with control and exhale to repeat.

HOW MANY DO I DO?
Perform 5 reps

Lengthen the thighs as you lift

Scoop the abs

Press the arms firmly down

Curl the tailbone up

Keep the feet flat

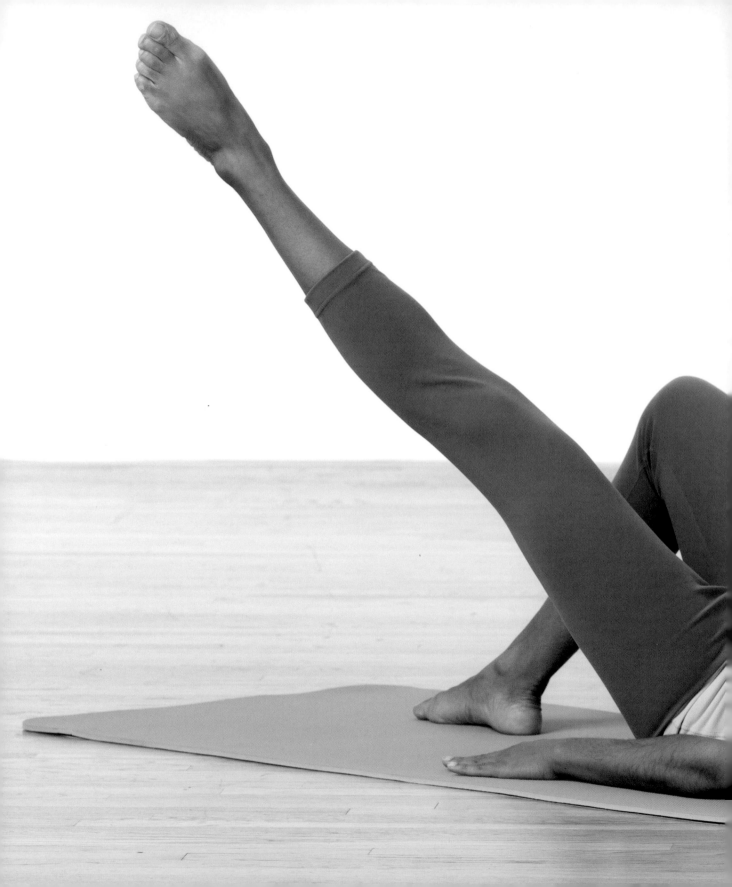

Beginner

Everyone's a beginner when they start Pilates.
If you're an experienced exerciser, you'll find
this is a whole new way to move your body.
For new exercisers, take your time and enjoy
the improved body you're about to create.

Centring
Focus on centring

No Pilates practice can begin without first learning how to move from your centre. Master this move and then come back to it over and over again to reinforce the sensation of initiating from your powerhouse (see p.61).

1 Lie on your back with your knees bent and your feet flat. Take a few breaths and let your body sink comfortably into the mat.

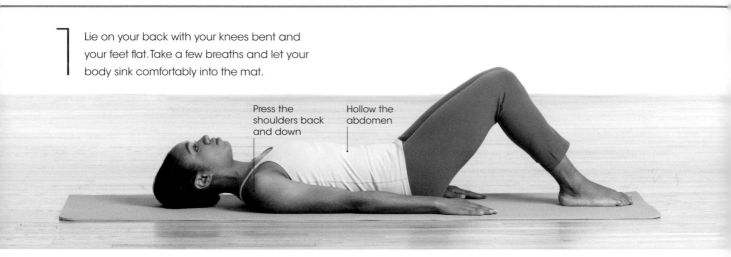

Press the shoulders back and down

Hollow the abdomen

2 Simultaneously stretch one arm back and the opposite leg forward. Focus on keeping your spine solid. Try not to arch or hunch your back. Slide your arm and leg back to your starting position. Repeat on the other side.

HOW MANY DO I DO?
Alternate for 5–8 sets

TEMPO
Slow

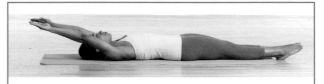

Ready for a challenge?
Try stretching both arms and both legs at the same time. Hold strong in your core (see p.61) throughout.

Anchor the torso

Stretch the leg long

Keep the back solid

Neck Peel
Focus on precision

Flat-ab seekers suffer with sore necks all the time. Grab an exercise band and practise peeling your neck from the floor just as you would peel a banana. Use the band to help you work in a smooth, controlled and deliberate manner.

1 Lie flat on your back on top of a band or towel. Make sure the band is centred down the middle of your spine. Bend both knees and take hold of the band above your head.

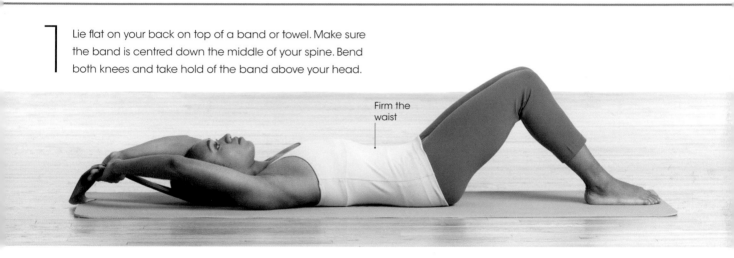

Firm the waist

2 Gently peel your body up, initiating the movement from your abs. Let your head be heavy so that your tummy does all the work. Stop at the peak of the curl and take a breath. Exhale to return slowly to the mat.

HOW MANY DO I DO?
Perform 5 reps, contracting the abs deeper with each rep

TEMPO
Slow

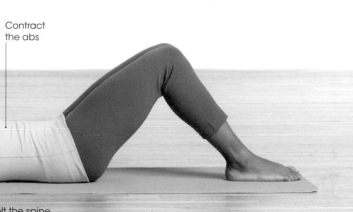

Hold the band with both hands

Keep the neck long with space under the chin

Contract the abs

Melt the spine into the mat

Hundred Prep
Focus on breath

I use this version with students who have difficulty accessing their deep abdominal muscles. Do two full sets of 50 to pump up your lungs and set your heart rate for the rest of your workout. This will be your warm-up. When you've finished, you should be slightly breathless.

1 Sit up tall with your knees bent and hold behind your knees. Open your elbows to the sides and scoop your tummy in and up (see p.61). Take a breath to begin, then start curling down back towards the mat.

Curl the lower back from this point

Curl the hips under

2 Go as low as you can, curling your hips under you. Keep your upper back and shoulders in the air, but press your lower back firmly into the mat. Keeping your body at that level, release your hands to your sides.

Open the elbows wide

Hold behind the thighs

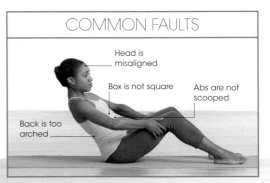

COMMON FAULTS

Head is misaligned

Box is not square

Abs are not scooped

Back is too arched

3 Begin to pump your arms energetically up and down, inhaling for 5 pumps then exhaling for 5 pumps until you reach 50. Sit up to begin again, then roll down a bit lower. Release your arms and pump up and down once more for a second set of 50. Pause at the end to scoop your abs, take hold of your legs and exhale to round back up to a sitting position.

HOW MANY DO I DO?
Perform 2 x 50 pumps or
1 x 100 pumps

TEMPO
Rapid

Ready for a challenge?
Do just one set, pumping all the way to 100.

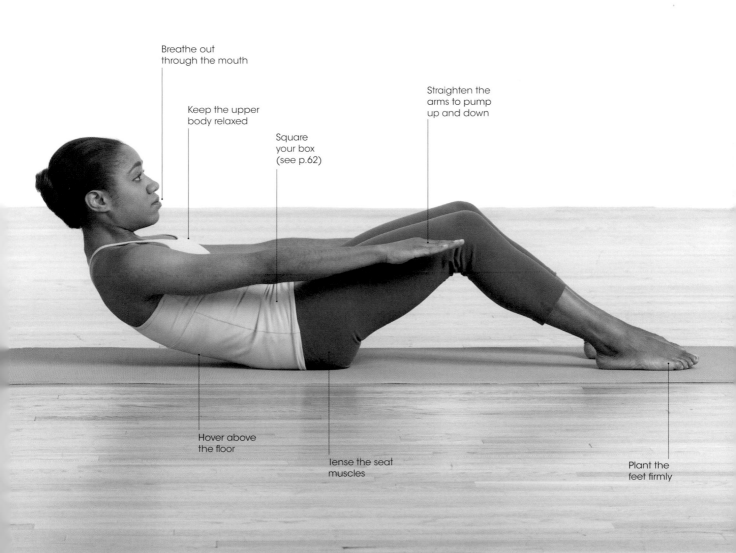

Breathe out
through the mouth

Keep the upper
body relaxed

Square
your box
(see p.62)

Straighten the
arms to pump
up and down

Hover above
the floor

Tense the seat
muscles

Plant the
feet firmly

Roll-Back
Focus on centring

Your lower back and abdominals will be eternally grateful for this exercise. Students can sometimes get stuck at one level, so be sure to go lower each time you repeat the move, challenging your core as well as your control.

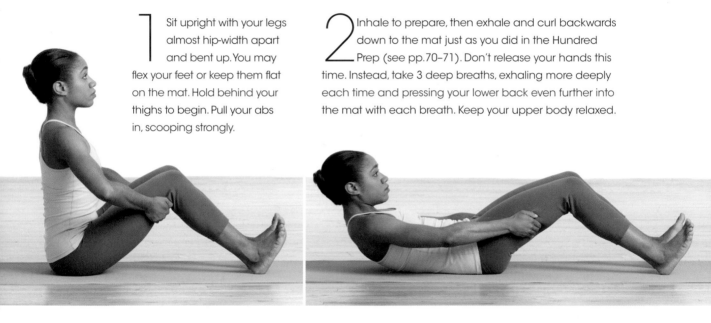

1 Sit upright with your legs almost hip-width apart and bent up. You may flex your feet or keep them flat on the mat. Hold behind your thighs to begin. Pull your abs in, scooping strongly.

2 Inhale to prepare, then exhale and curl backwards down to the mat just as you did in the Hundred Prep (see pp.70–71). Don't release your hands this time. Instead, take 3 deep breaths, exhaling more deeply each time and pressing your lower back even further into the mat with each breath. Keep your upper body relaxed.

3 On the third breath, round back over your legs, pulling back in your abs as though you were resisting coming forward. Sit up tall to begin again.

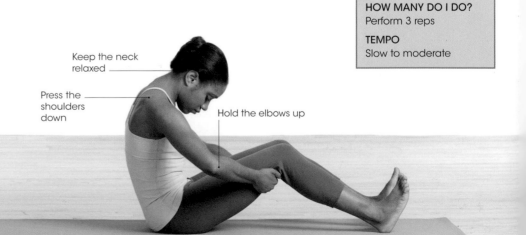

Keep the neck relaxed

Press the shoulders down

Hold the elbows up

HOW MANY DO I DO?
Perform 3 reps

TEMPO
Slow to moderate

Roll-Up
Focus on control

Up and over. Back and down. It's just that simple. Become your own instructor by repeating the directions to yourself as you work out. Keep your movements fluid and rhythmical as you tackle the first proper sit-up in the Beginner programme.

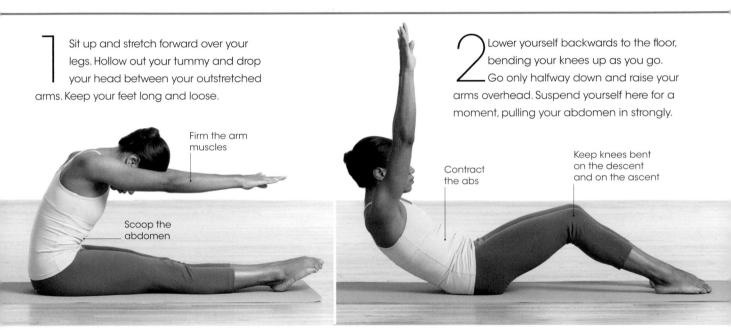

1 Sit up and stretch forward over your legs. Hollow out your tummy and drop your head between your outstretched arms. Keep your feet long and loose.

Firm the arm muscles

Scoop the abdomen

2 Lower yourself backwards to the floor, bending your knees up as you go. Go only halfway down and raise your arms overhead. Suspend yourself here for a moment, pulling your abdomen in strongly.

Contract the abs

Keep knees bent on the descent and on the ascent

3 Lower your arms and exhale to begin curling up and over. Keep your knees bent as you come up to sitting, then straighten your legs as you round your body over to return to the Step 1 position.

HOW MANY DO I DO?
Perform 6–8 reps, becoming more fluid with each rep

TEMPO
Moderate

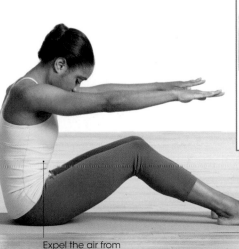

Expel the air from the abdomen

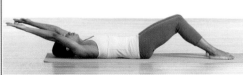

Ready for a challenge?
Lower yourself to the floor, stretching your arms all the way back. Use your powerhouse to fold back up without using momentum.

Leg Circles
Focus on precision

Circling your leg in the air is not hard. Doing it precisely and correctly without letting your body twist round is a completely different story. Use this move to reinforce your basic principles. Anchor your powerhouse and hold your body strong and steady.

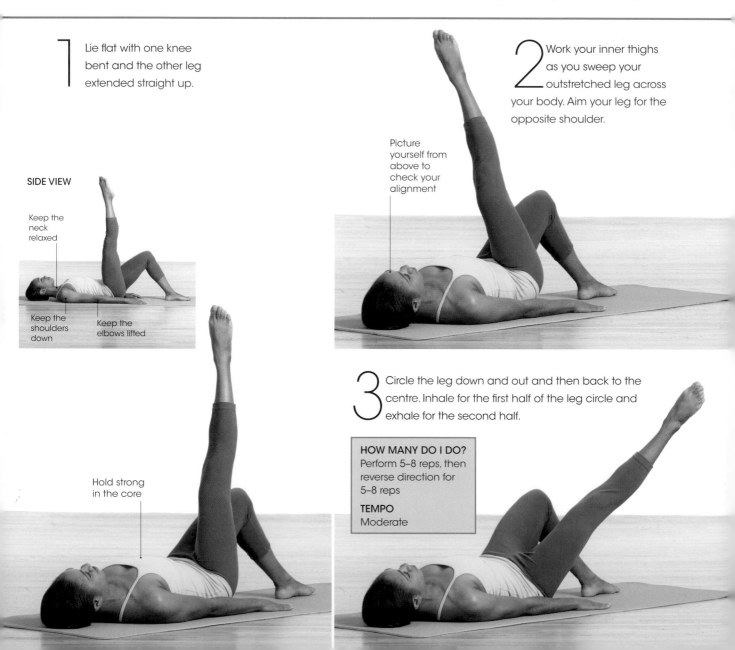

1 Lie flat with one knee bent and the other leg extended straight up.

SIDE VIEW

Keep the neck relaxed

Keep the shoulders down

Keep the elbows lifted

Hold strong in the core

2 Work your inner thighs as you sweep your outstretched leg across your body. Aim your leg for the opposite shoulder.

Picture yourself from above to check your alignment

3 Circle the leg down and out and then back to the centre. Inhale for the first half of the leg circle and exhale for the second half.

HOW MANY DO I DO?
Perform 5–8 reps, then reverse direction for 5–8 reps

TEMPO
Moderate

Rolling Like a Ball I

Focus on concentration

Timing is everything in the Pilates method. Rolling Like a Ball I can be done quickly or slowly. Do it quickly if you are working on flow and rhythm, but practise more slowly to develop your strength and control.

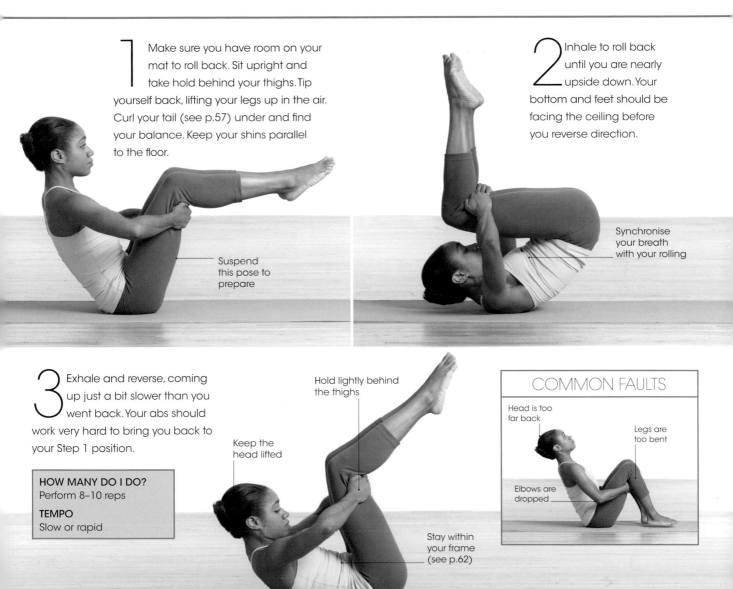

1 Make sure you have room on your mat to roll back. Sit upright and take hold behind your thighs. Tip yourself back, lifting your legs up in the air. Curl your tail (see p.57) under and find your balance. Keep your shins parallel to the floor.

Suspend this pose to prepare

2 Inhale to roll back until you are nearly upside down. Your bottom and feet should be facing the ceiling before you reverse direction.

Synchronise your breath with your rolling

3 Exhale and reverse, coming up just a bit slower than you went back. Your abs should work very hard to bring you back to your Step 1 position.

HOW MANY DO I DO?
Perform 8–10 reps

TEMPO
Slow or rapid

Hold lightly behind the thighs

Keep the head lifted

Stay within your frame (see p.62)

COMMON FAULTS

Head is too far back

Legs are too bent

Elbows are dropped

Single Leg Stretch I
Focus on centring

The name implies a stretching move, but Single Leg Stretch I is so much more. Your alignment is key to your success here. Be sure not to pose or pause just to be properly placed, but move rhythmically and with energy.

1 From a lying-down position, inhale as you lift your head and shoulders and hug your right leg into your chest. At the same time, stretch your left leg out long and take it towards the centre line of your body (see p.57). Contract your glutes as you extend your leg.

Lengthen the leg

Keep the elbows wide

Tighten the glutes

2 Exhale as you switch to the other leg, then continue alternating, slowly at first, but gradually reaching a moderate speed. Always inhale when you extend your left leg and exhale when you extend your right leg.

Layer the hands over the knee

HOW MANY DO I DO?
Alternate for 8 sets

TEMPO
Slow to moderate

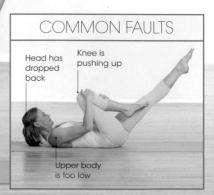

COMMON FAULTS

Head has dropped back

Knee is pushing up

Upper body is too low

Double Leg Stretch I
Focus on control

Remember the Centring exercise (see p.68), where you learned to initiate from the core and lengthen your limbs fully. Double Leg Stretch I will reinforce that habit and strengthen your overall Pilates practice.

1 Lie on your back and hug both knees in tight to your body. Using your abs, lift your head to meet your knees.

2 Keep your head up and your abs in as you inhale and stretch your arms forward.

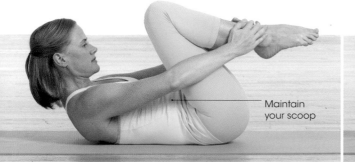

Maintain your scoop

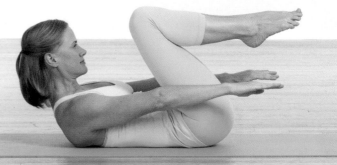

3 Extend your legs forward. Draw your abs in one last time and then exhale as you bend your knees back in. Hug your knees tight and repeat. Always inhale to extend and exhale to fold back in.

HOW MANY DO I DO?
Perform 6–8 reps

TEMPO
Slow to moderate

Ready for a challenge?
As you get stronger, try taking your legs lower and curl up even higher.

Sink the abs deeper as the limbs stretch out

Keep the head and shoulders lifted as the limbs extend

Keep the back flat on the mat

Spine Stretch Forward I
Focus on breath

Now you'll put your C-curve (see p.63) to work. This version of Spine Stretch Forward borrows from one of Mr Pilates' students, Carola Trier. Use this move to improve your posture and flexibility at the same time as you are working your core.

1 Sit up with your legs astride your mat and your hands between your legs, pressing down into the mat. Use the downward pressure of your arms to lift your torso higher and longer and give you good posture.

Plant the hands firmly down

Square your box to sit tall

2 Inhale, then exhale as you slide your hands forward on the floor, rounding forward to take hold of the arches of your feet. Resist in your waist as you gently tug yourself forward. Release your hands and slide back up tall and straight, once again pressing your palms firmly into the floor.

HOW MANY DO I DO?
Perform 5 reps
TEMPO
Slow

Keep the neck long

Keep the shoulders down

Pull back in the waist as you round forward

Take hold of the ankles

Spine Twist I
Focus on precision

Depending on how you feel, you can use Spine Twist I as a stretching move or a strengthening move. Either way, you'll need your very best posture (see pp.20–21) and good torso control.

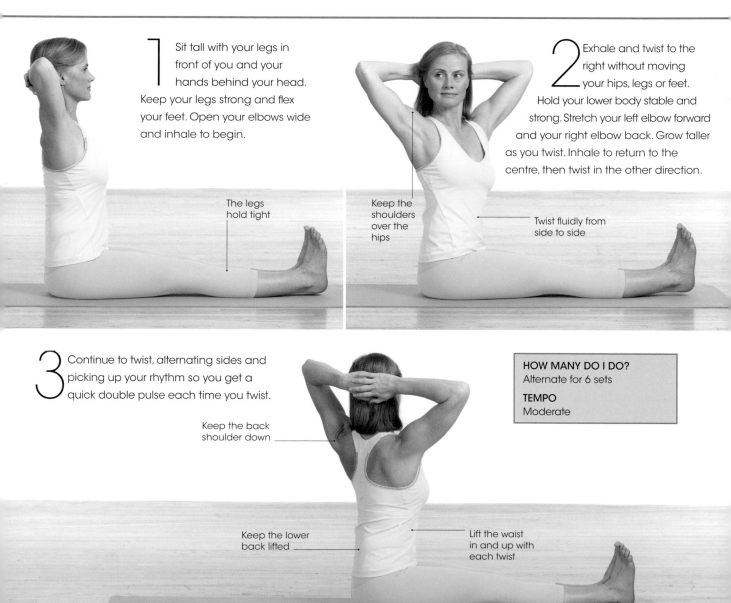

1 Sit tall with your legs in front of you and your hands behind your head. Keep your legs strong and flex your feet. Open your elbows wide and inhale to begin.

The legs hold tight

2 Exhale and twist to the right without moving your hips, legs or feet. Hold your lower body stable and strong. Stretch your left elbow forward and your right elbow back. Grow taller as you twist. Inhale to return to the centre, then twist in the other direction.

Keep the shoulders over the hips

Twist fluidly from side to side

3 Continue to twist, alternating sides and picking up your rhythm so you get a quick double pulse each time you twist.

Keep the back shoulder down

HOW MANY DO I DO?
Alternate for 6 sets

TEMPO
Moderate

Keep the lower back lifted

Lift the waist in and up with each twist

Bottom Walk
Focus on flow

Bottom Walk was taught to me years ago and is rarely included in the traditional Pilates vocabulary. Have some fun with this move and tone your bottom, strengthen your hips and develop your balance and coordination at the same time.

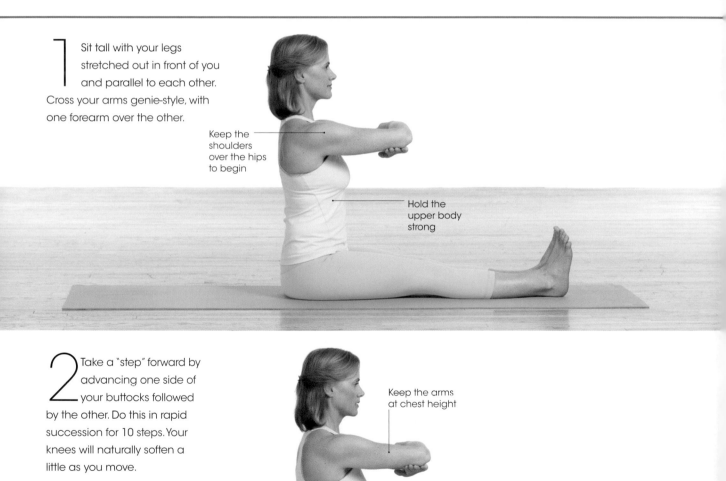

1 Sit tall with your legs stretched out in front of you and parallel to each other. Cross your arms genie-style, with one forearm over the other.

Keep the shoulders over the hips to begin

Hold the upper body strong

2 Take a "step" forward by advancing one side of your buttocks followed by the other. Do this in rapid succession for 10 steps. Your knees will naturally soften a little as you move.

Keep the arms at chest height

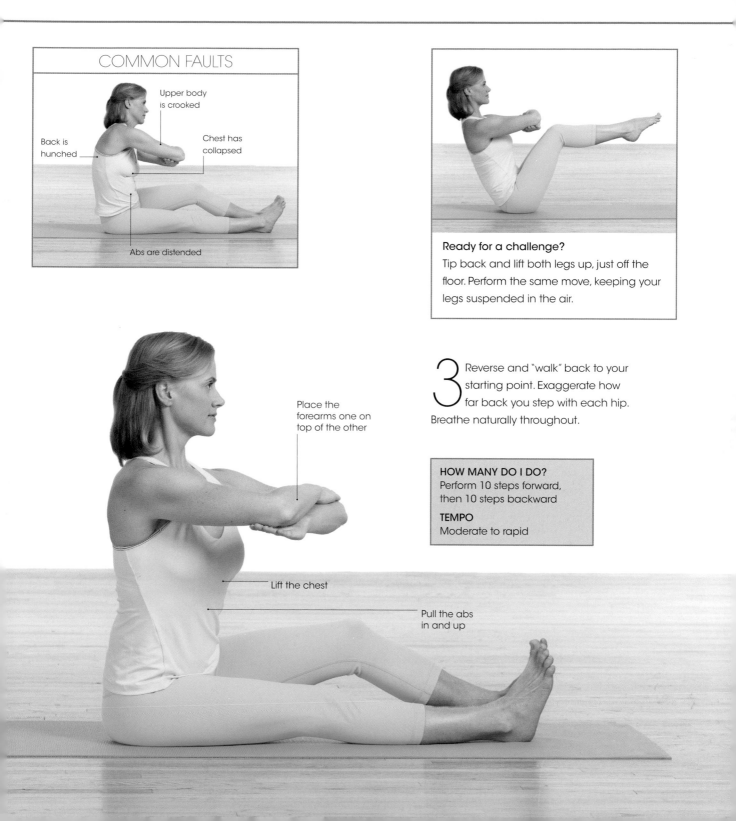

COMMON FAULTS

Upper body is crooked

Back is hunched

Chest has collapsed

Abs are distended

Ready for a challenge?
Tip back and lift both legs up, just off the floor. Perform the same move, keeping your legs suspended in the air.

3 Reverse and "walk" back to your starting point. Exaggerate how far back you step with each hip. Breathe naturally throughout.

HOW MANY DO I DO?
Perform 10 steps forward, then 10 steps backward

TEMPO
Moderate to rapid

Place the forearms one on top of the other

Lift the chest

Pull the abs in and up

Tick-Tock
Focus on control

Your waist will thank you for Tick-Tock. Take this one slowly and be sure that your abdominals don't cheat by pushing out, away from the body. Begin with small motions and gradually make the move larger, like the pendulum on a grandfather clock.

1 Lie flat with your legs straight up at 90°. Spread your arms out to the sides and press them into the floor. Inhale to prepare.

2 Inhale and lower both legs over to your right side. Reach them away from your body and keep them as straight as possible. As your legs move to the right, pull your left hip down in opposition. Keep your arms pressed into the floor throughout. Exhale and bring your legs back to the centre line, then repeat, lowering your legs to the left.

OPPOSITE SIDE

HOW MANY DO I DO?
Alternate for 4–5 sets

TEMPO
Slow

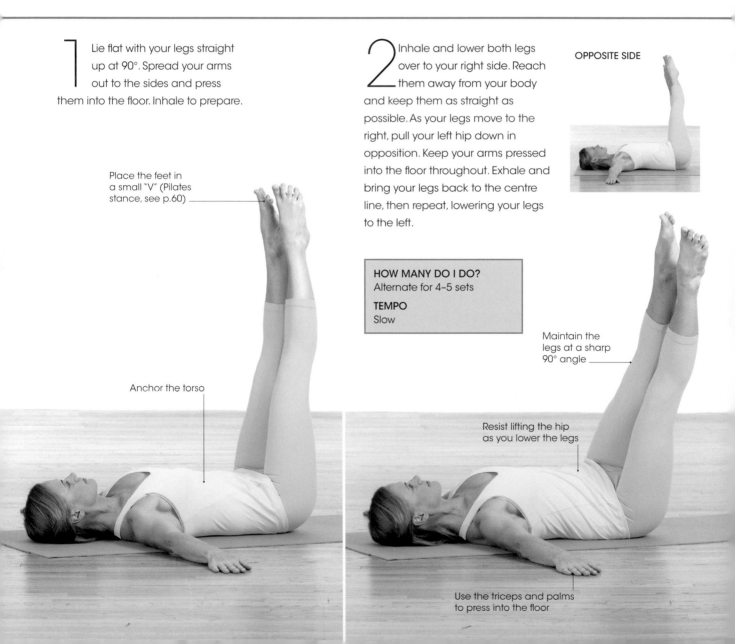

Place the feet in a small "V" (Pilates stance, see p.60)

Anchor the torso

Maintain the legs at a sharp 90° angle

Resist lifting the hip as you lower the legs

Use the triceps and palms to press into the floor

Swan Prep
Focus on precision

I call this the gravity-fighter exercise. All day long, gravity is pushing down on your skeleton. Here's your chance to fight back. This simple move is one I recommend you perform when you don't have time for anything else.

1 Lie on your stomach with your legs together. Place your hands precisely under your shoulders and draw your upper arms in tight to your body so your elbows point straight back.

Squeeze the elbows in towards the body

Firm the leg muscles

2 Press your upper body up 10–15cm (4–6in) from the floor, lifting your head and chest to look straight ahead. Hover there for 5 breaths, pulling up your abs and opening your chest. Contract your upper-back muscles as though you were squeezing your shoulder blades together. Lower yourself slowly with control.

HOW MANY DO I DO?
Perform 3–5 reps

TEMPO
Slow

Press the shoulders down

Keep the legs as close together as possible

Lift the chest

Knee Stretches
Focus on centring

Practise your coordination and mobilise your spine with this exercise borrowed from the Pilates Reformer machine (see p.217). Exaggerate this movement as you round up and under. Start slowly and pick up speed as you increase your control.

1 Kneel on all fours on your mat. Place your hands under your shoulders and your knees under your hips. Make sure your spine is completely flat and keep your neck long.

2 Exhale and round your back, dropping your head and hips downwards. At the same time, lift your right knee and pull it under you, aiming your knee towards your forehead.

3 Inhale and stretch your right leg out behind you, lifting your head and extending your spine. Keep your abs working and your hips square.

HOW MANY DO I DO?
Perform 5–8 reps, then switch sides for 5–8 reps

TEMPO
Moderate

Lengthen the leg away from the body

Keep the shoulders square

Work the abs

Side Kicks: Front I
Focus on control

This exercise is the only one of the Side Kicks Series shown by Mr Pilates in his book *Return to Life.* In this book, you'll learn many variations. Be sure to complete all the Side Kicks in your programme (see also pp.86 and 87) on one side before switching sides.

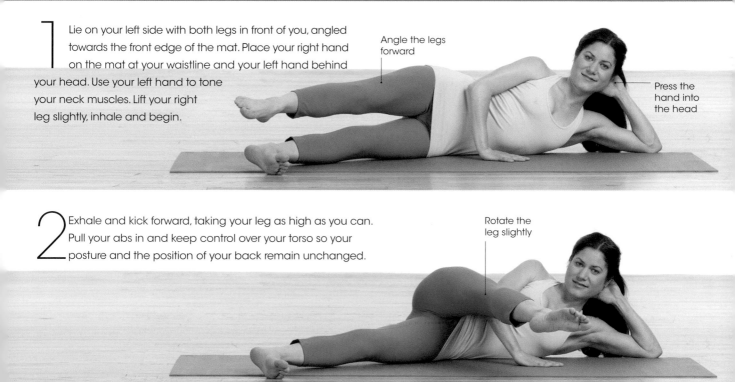

1 Lie on your left side with both legs in front of you, angled towards the front edge of the mat. Place your right hand on the mat at your waistline and your left hand behind your head. Use your left hand to tone your neck muscles. Lift your right leg slightly, inhale and begin.

Angle the legs forward

Press the hand into the head

2 Exhale and kick forward, taking your leg as high as you can. Pull your abs in and keep control over your torso so your posture and the position of your back remain unchanged.

Rotate the leg slightly

3 Without leaning forward, breathe in with the air and kick back, swinging your leg as far back as you can.

Keep the kicking leg straight

Lengthen the lower back

HOW MANY DO I DO?
Perform 8 reps. Repeat on each side.

TEMPO
Moderate

Side Kicks: Double Leg Lift
Focus on precision

Building on Side Kicks: Front (see p.85), this variation is meant to wake up your lateral, or side, muscles. These help to keep you upright. You will still be working your legs but this move will challenge your balance and timing as well as your muscles.

1 Lie on your left side as for Side Kicks: Front (see p.85). Place your right hand on the mat in front of your abs for support. Be sure your upper body is against the back edge of the mat and your feet reach the front edge.

Maintain tension between the head and hand

Activate the glutes to rotate the legs

Press heel to heel

2 With one solid movement, lift both legs, squeezing them together tightly. Pause in the air for a moment, then set them down lightly. Breathe naturally throughout. As you gain mobility, lift your legs higher with each repetition.

HOW MANY DO I DO?
Perform 5 reps.
Repeat on each side.

TEMPO
Moderate

Relax the neck

Compress the leg muscles

Stack the shoulders and hips

Press the shoulders down

Keep the legs at an angle

Side Kicks: Lower Lift
Focus on concentration

To perform the "lower and lift", you'll need a strong core, good balance and a bit of coordination. Remember that all muscles work all the time in Pilates. When you've finished, flip onto your other side and start the Side Kicks all over again from p.85.

1 Lie on your left side with your right hand on the mat in front of you as for Side Kicks: Front (see p.85). Position your legs in front of you, angled forward. Exhale as you lift both legs, holding them tightly together.

STARTING POSITION

Keep the legs angled forward

Maintain the Pilates stance

Keep the arm muscles relaxed

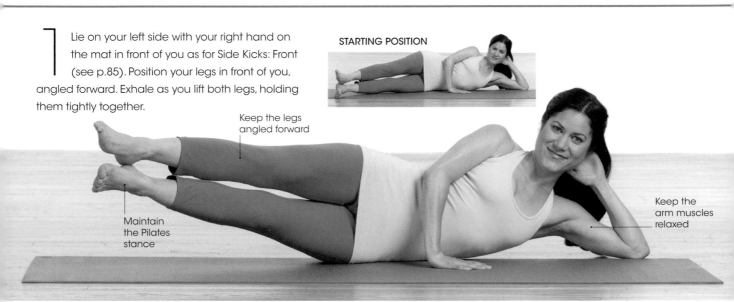

2 From this position, inhale as you lower your left leg to just above the floor, then exhale as you lift it back up. Use your inner-thigh muscles as you continue lowering and lifting your leg. Coordinate your breathing so that each time your leg lifts, you actively exhale.

HOW MANY DO I DO?
Perform 8 reps.
Repeat on each side.

TEMPO
Moderate

Relax the upper body

Suspend the lower leg in the air

Maintain resistance between the head and the hand

Mermaid

Focus on flow

One of my favourite moves in the Pilates vocabulary, Mermaid is performed in many variations in studios worldwide. This particular exercise works the often-neglected sides of the body that are difficult to target in other exercises.

1 Sit to the right side of your legs with your knees and feet tucked in tight to your body. Reach your left hand down to the bottom ankle to hold of it. Stack your legs with your knees, shins and feet together, one leg over the other. Extend your right arm straight up and press it alongside your head.

2 Exhale fully as you reach up and to the left over your legs, bending at your waist. Try to reach up rather than bend down so that your waist extends.

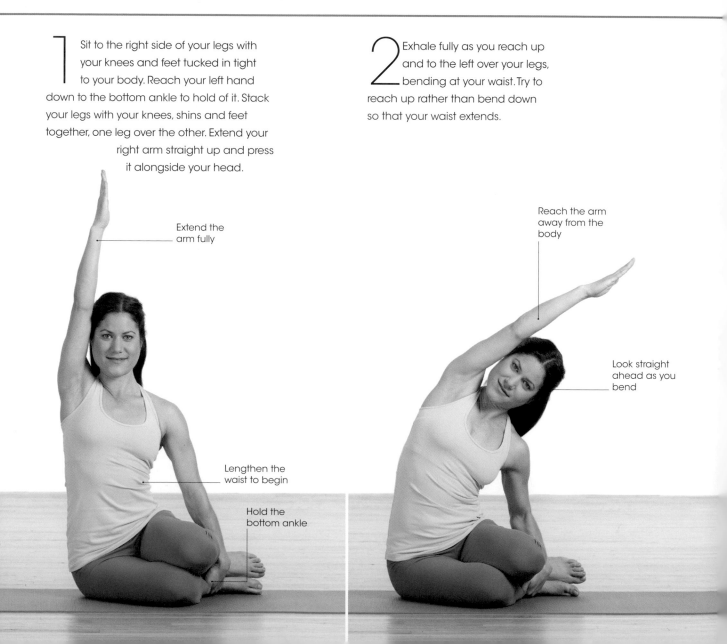

Extend the arm fully

Lengthen the waist to begin

Hold the bottom ankle

Reach the arm away from the body

Look straight ahead as you bend

3 Inhale as you return to an upright position. Release your ankles and float your left arm up, then exhale fully as you stretch the other way, taking your right hand to the floor and keeping your arm straight.

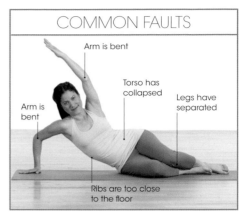

COMMON FAULTS

Arm is bent

Torso has collapsed

Legs have separated

Arm is bent

Ribs are too close to the floor

Be strong in the waist to support your weight

4 Spring your right hand up off the floor to return to an upright position to begin again. As you repeat, go lower each time in both directions. With each repetition, push more strongly off the floor.

HOW MANY DO I DO?
Perform 3–5 reps, then switch sides for 3–5 reps

TEMPO
Moderate

Press the shoulder down

Keep the ribcage lifted

Shoulder Bridge
Focus on control

Here's a move that builds stamina as well as strength. This is a hybrid move I use routinely to challenge the back of the body. Mr Pilates was influenced by yoga, and Shoulder Bridge clearly demonstrates those early influences.

1 Lie flat on your back with your knees bent and your arms by your sides. Ensure your feet and knees are hip-width apart. Keep your feet flat on the mat.

Keep the knees hip-width apart

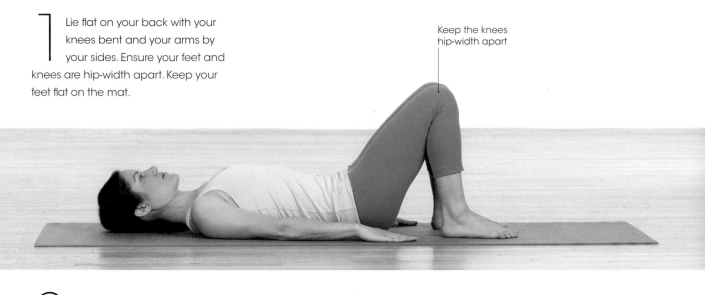

2 Inhale, then exhale as you raise your hips. Keep your upper body firm, holding your ribs in to avoid arching. Contract your buttocks and hamstrings strongly. Hold for 5 breaths. You may lower here or continue to Step 3 if you are ready.

Hold one long line from head to knees

Drive the hips up strongly

Keep the feet directly under the knees

Work the triceps

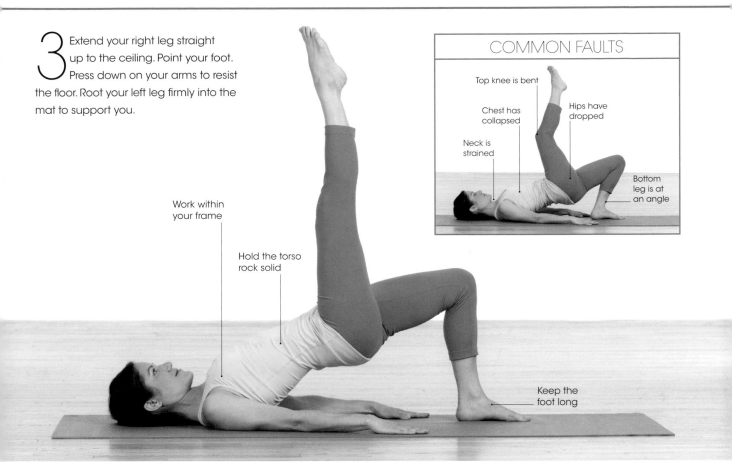

3 Extend your right leg straight up to the ceiling. Point your foot. Press down on your arms to resist the floor. Root your left leg firmly into the mat to support you.

Work within your frame

Hold the torso rock solid

Keep the foot long

COMMON FAULTS

Top knee is bent

Chest has collapsed

Hips have dropped

Neck is strained

Bottom leg is at an angle

4 Inhale as you kick your leg down and flex your foot. Continue kicking up and pointing, then kicking down and flexing. Time your breathing so that you exhale on every upward kick. Replace your right leg on the mat and repeat with your left leg. Finish by replacing both feet and rolling down through your spine to the mat.

HOW MANY DO I DO?
Perform 5 reps, then switch sides for 5 reps

TEMPO
Moderate to rapid

Keep the hips high

Suspend the foot above the mat

Keep the heel forward as you kick down

Windmill
Focus on breath

Windmill was introduced by Mr Pilates using a device called the Breath-a-Cizer (see p.47). The Pilates Elders – Mr Pilates' original students – all have a different approach to the use of the breath in Pilates, but this exercise has remained in the Pilates archives.

1 Stand tall with your best posture, hands placed behind your head. Imagine a plumb line running from your ear down your shoulder, hip and ankle. With your skeleton aligned, inhale to begin.

2 Begin a slow exhale and start to roll down from the top of your head. Allow the weight of your head to pull you forward and down as you lift in and up in the waistline. You have reached the bottom of the roll when you have no more air left to exhale.

3 Slowly inhale to roll back up to standing, one vertebra at a time. Stack each vertebra on top of the one below it. As you come to an upright position, roll your shoulders back and bring your head up to your starting position.

HOW MANY DO I DO?
Perform 3 reps

TEMPO
Slow

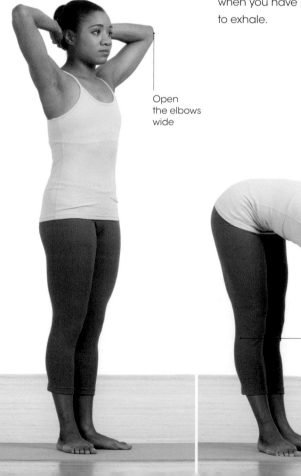

Open the elbows wide

Sink the upper body down

Press the backs of the legs together

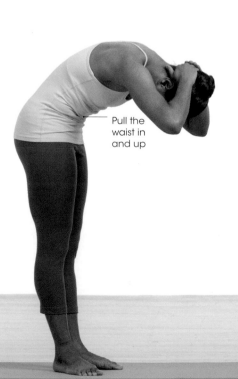

Pull the waist in and up

Front Curls
Focus on centring

If this were solely an arm exercise, I would suggest more weight. But Pilates works all muscles all the time. Use the weight most appropriate to your body. I suggest 0.5–2kg (2–5lb) weights to get the most out of it. Use resistance the entire time.

1 Stand tall with your legs together and your feet in Pilates stance. Tense your buttocks, lift your abs and hold strong in your torso. Take your arms in front of you, directly in line with your shoulders. Lean forward slightly to counter any tendency to lean back.

2 Inhale as you bend at your elbows and fold your arms in past 90° but no farther than your temples. Actively exhale as you extend your arms again, resisting as you do so. When you have completed all your reps, lower your arms to finish.

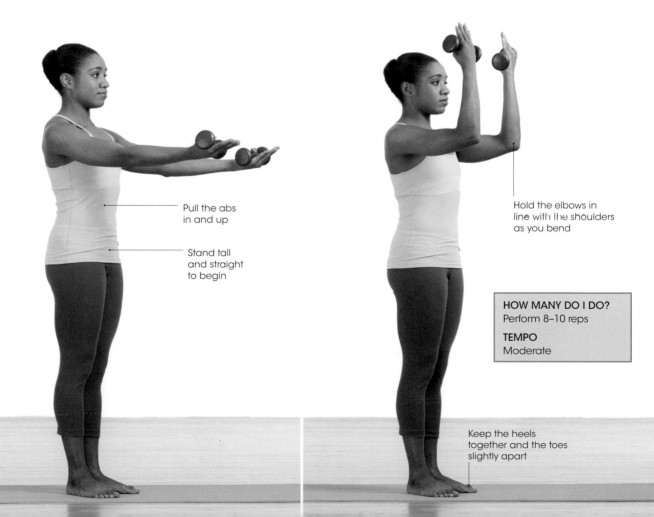

Pull the abs in and up

Stand tall and straight to begin

Hold the elbows in line with the shoulders as you bend

HOW MANY DO I DO?
Perform 8–10 reps

TEMPO
Moderate

Keep the heels together and the toes slightly apart

Side Curls
Focus on precision

Move from Front Curls into Side Curls to target your arm muscles from a different direction. This move is second in a series of exercises with weights, so stand even straighter and taller to combat the fatigue you will be feeling in your arms.

1 Raise your arms out to the sides but keep them within your peripheral vision. Keep your arms and wrists straight. Tense your buttock muscles and tighten your waistline as you inhale to begin.

2 Bend your arms in towards your head, folding them past 90° and aiming for your temples. Exhale and resist the motion as you extend your arms again. When you have completed all your reps, lower your arms to finish.

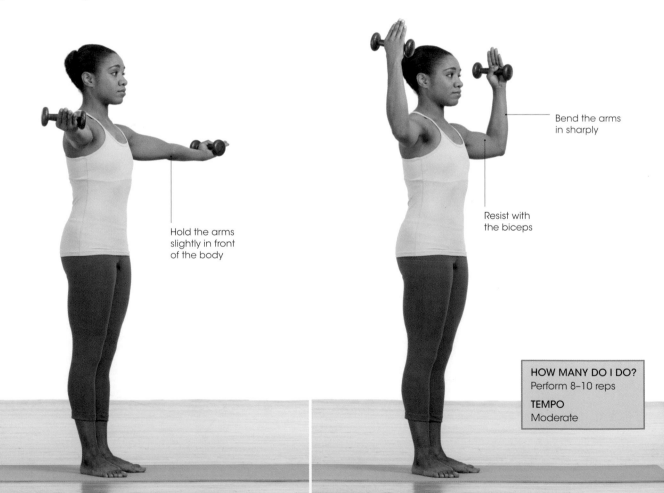

Hold the arms slightly in front of the body

Bend the arms in sharply

Resist with the biceps

HOW MANY DO I DO?
Perform 8–10 reps

TEMPO
Moderate

Sparklers
Focus on control

Named for the fireworks that you hold in your hand, Sparklers gives you a strong visual image to work with. As you work through the move, just imagine the design you would make in the air if you were holding real sparklers.

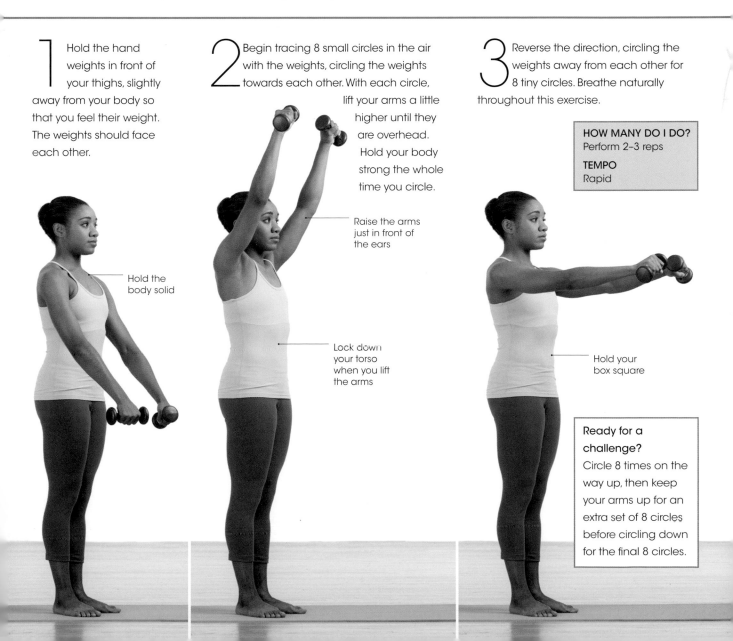

1 Hold the hand weights in front of your thighs, slightly away from your body so that you feel their weight. The weights should face each other.

Hold the body solid

2 Begin tracing 8 small circles in the air with the weights, circling the weights towards each other. With each circle, lift your arms a little higher until they are overhead. Hold your body strong the whole time you circle.

Raise the arms just in front of the ears

Lock down your torso when you lift the arms

3 Reverse the direction, circling the weights away from each other for 8 tiny circles. Breathe naturally throughout this exercise.

HOW MANY DO I DO?
Perform 2–3 reps

TEMPO
Rapid

Hold your box square

Ready for a challenge?
Circle 8 times on the way up, then keep your arms up for an extra set of 8 circles before circling down for the final 8 circles.

Wall: Stand
Focus on breath

Poor posture is responsible for many muscular and skeletal disorders. This simple move, that you can do anywhere at any time, is a perfect way to keep your posture in check. Even if a full workout isn't possible, this move is always an option.

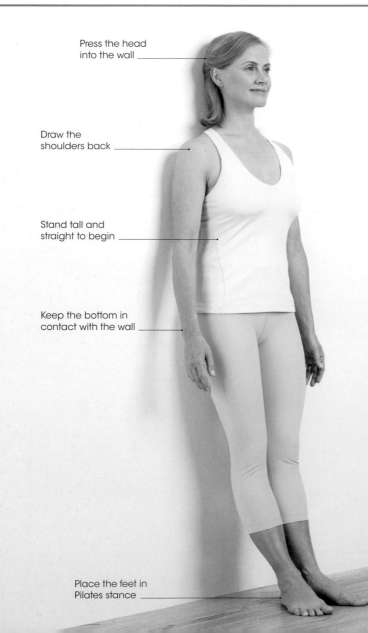

Press the head into the wall

Draw the shoulders back

Stand tall and straight to begin

Keep the bottom in contact with the wall

Place the feet in Pilates stance

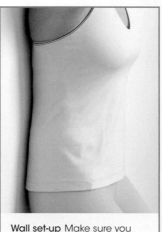

Wall set-up Make sure you can fully lengthen your spine against the wall. Keep your bottom against the wall so as not to tuck under.

Stand at the wall with your back firmly against it from the back of your head down to your tail. Place your feet one step in front of you so that you are leaning into the wall. Stand still for 5–10 breaths, making tiny adjustments to keep your neck long, your shoulders down, your chest high, your ribs in and your lower back long. Breathe fully and deeply.

Ready for a challenge?
Hold a set of small hand weights when doing this move and Wall: Circles (see opposite).

Wall: Circles
Focus on centring

Use this move to build on the posture work you did in Wall: Stand (see opposite). Adding mobility to a static pose can be tricky. Continue to work on the basics of Wall: Stand, but don't sacrifice any of the details as you practise this variation.

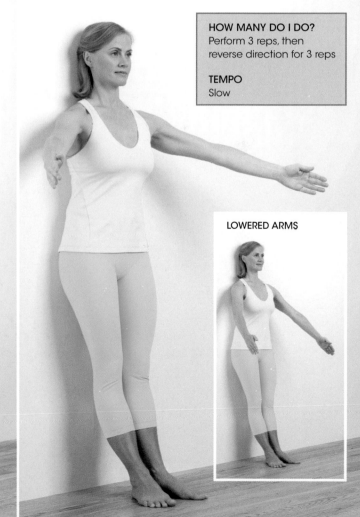

Keep the shoulders in contact with the wall

Keep the ribs still

Place the feet in Pilates stance

1 Stand as for Wall: Stand (see opposite). If necessary, bend your legs slightly in order to lengthen your lower back. Draw your abs in. Raise your arms in front of you then up overhead to begin a big arm circle. At the peak of the circle, exhale to draw your abs even tighter and higher. Do not disturb the alignment of your spine against the wall.

2 Open your arms out to the sides, but keep them within your peripheral vision as you lower them back down to the front of your body.

HOW MANY DO I DO?
Perform 3 reps, then reverse direction for 3 reps

TEMPO
Slow

LOWERED ARMS

Wall: Chair
Focus on concentration

Whether you exercise once in a blue moon or every day, Wall: Chair is uniquely effective. By now, control and precision are second nature. In addition to that, this exercise challenges your endurance. Use your breath and a sharp mental focus.

1 Holding the hand weights, stand as for Wall: Stand (see p.96). Walk your feet a bit farther out and keep the legs parallel and hip-width apart.

Press the shoulders back

2 Bend your knees and slide down until it feels as if you are sitting in a chair. Your knees should be at 90°. Lift your arms to shoulder height. Hold for 5 breaths, working up to 10 breaths or 30 seconds. Press your heels firmly into the floor. Slide back up the wall and lower your arms to finish. To increase your stamina, practise holding for 1 full minute.

Keep the back in contact with the wall as you slide

HOW MANY DO I DO?
Perform 2 reps

TEMPO
Slow

Position the legs at 90°

Hold your position rock solid

Keep the heels flat

Two by Four

Focus on precision

Your feet hold you up all day long. Strengthen and align them with this move to improve their performance both while you exercise and in everyday life. Originally taught with a block of wood, this exercise is now performed on a level floor.

1 Stand braced against a wall with both feet flat and parallel. Your feet should be directly underneath you about two fists' distance apart. Bend your knees deeply to begin without allowing your heels to rise.

2 Keeping your knees bent, raise your heels as high as they will go. Transfer all your weight towards the front of your feet.

3 Squeeze your leg and glute muscles as you begin to straighten your legs. Resist any lowering of your heels as you straighten your legs. Pay close attention to your torso and powerhouse.

4 Slowly lower your heels. To reverse, rise up before bending your knees deeply. Then lower your heels and straighten up again. Breathe naturally.

HOW MANY DO I DO?
Perform 3 reps, then reverse direction for 3 reps

TEMPO
Slow to moderate

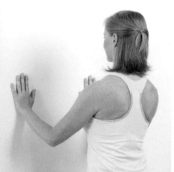

Keep the heels flat as the knees bend

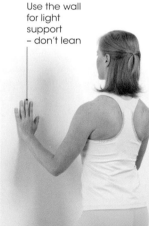

Use the wall for light support – don't lean

Keep the knees bent as you lift the heels

Focus the eyes ahead

Keep the upper body controlled but relaxed

Keep the knees directly over the toes

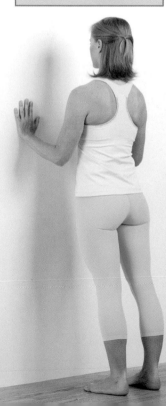

Front Splits
Focus on centring

Coupling deep stretches with alignment-based work is not easy. Front Splits offers both and will also challenge your balance. If your muscles begin to shake or quiver at any point, simply hold the position for three breaths and continue.

1 Bend into a deep lunge with your left leg forward. Take your hands to either side of your foot. Keep your right leg as straight as possible. Maintaining the position of your hands and feet, straighten and then bend your left leg 3 times. Exhale each time you straighten your leg.

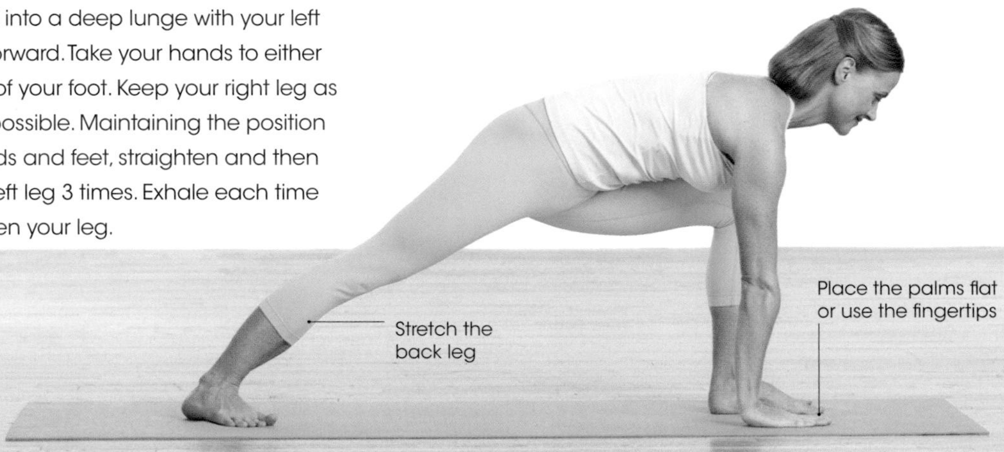

Stretch the back leg

Place the palms flat or use the fingertips

2 Find your balance, then cross your arms genie-style, forearm over forearm. Again without moving your hands or feet, stretch and bend your left leg 3 times, bending progressively deeper with each bend.

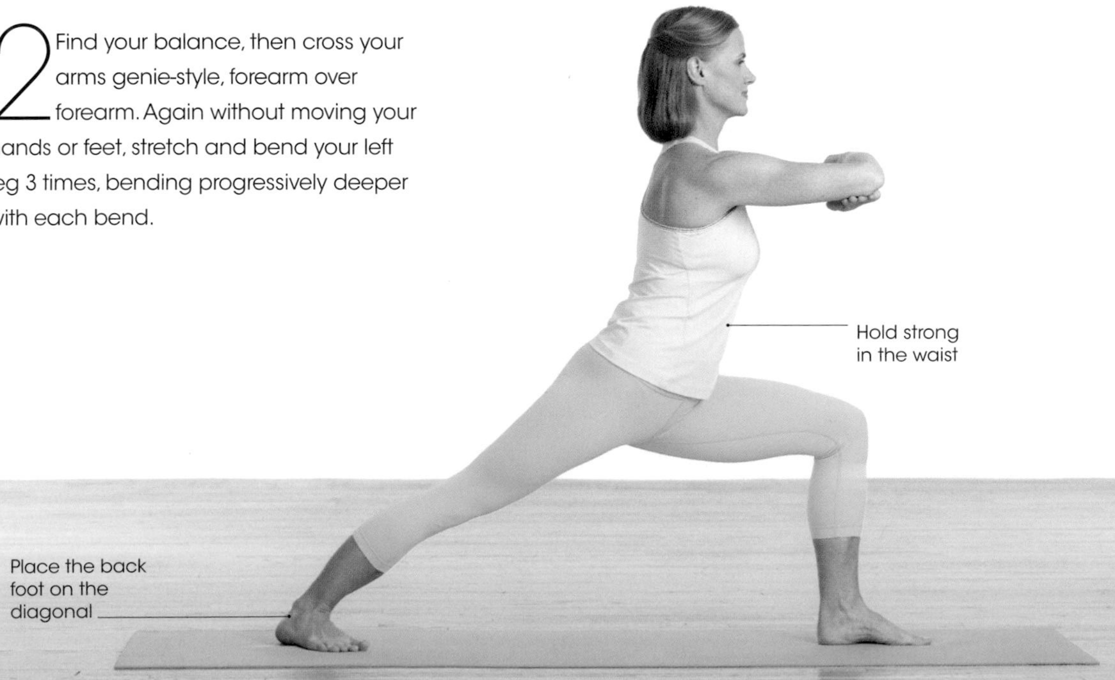

Hold strong in the waist

Place the back foot on the diagonal

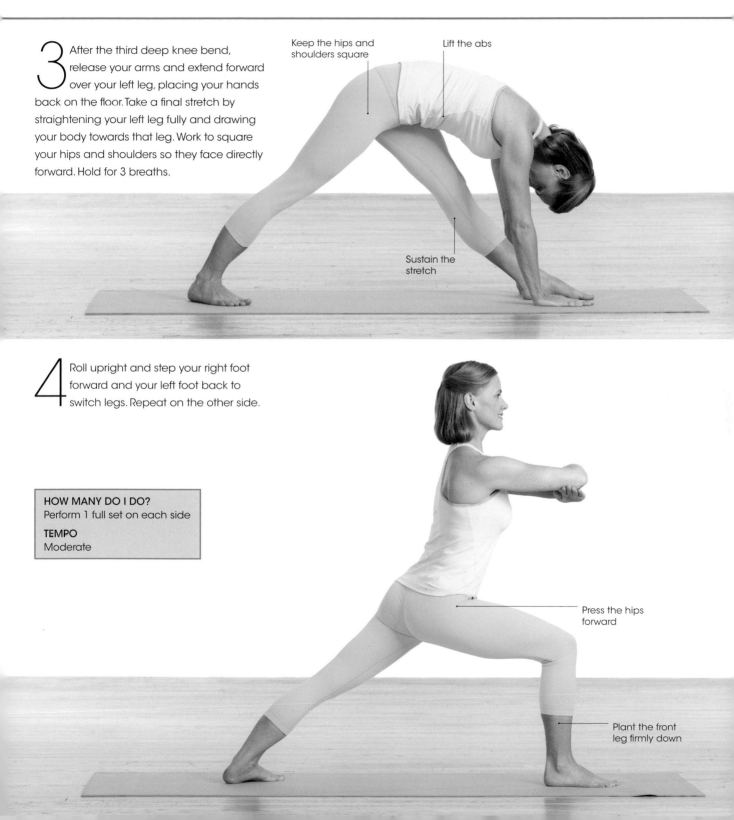

3 After the third deep knee bend, release your arms and extend forward over your left leg, placing your hands back on the floor. Take a final stretch by straightening your left leg fully and drawing your body towards that leg. Work to square your hips and shoulders so they face directly forward. Hold for 3 breaths.

Keep the hips and shoulders square

Lift the abs

Sustain the stretch

4 Roll upright and step your right foot forward and your left foot back to switch legs. Repeat on the other side.

HOW MANY DO I DO?
Perform 1 full set on each side

TEMPO
Moderate

Press the hips forward

Plant the front leg firmly down

Chest Expansion
Focus on breath

This move targets the opening and expanding of the chest, which yields a strengthening of the muscles of the upper back. Chest Expansion is a universal exercise, which means it is good for absolutely everyone.

1 Holding the hand weights, stand up tall with your feet in Pilates stance. Take both arms just in front of your body and slightly raised. Work your legs and buttocks by pressing them tightly together.

2 Inhale to begin, then press your arms back behind you. Expand your lungs, pull your shoulder blades in and keep your arms back.

3 Stretch your neck by turning your head left and then right. Return your head to the centre. Exhale as you float your arms back in front of you. Repeat, looking first to the left. With each set, open your chest more.

> **HOW MANY DO I DO?**
> Alternate for 3 sets
>
> **TEMPO**
> Moderate

Position the arms just in front of the legs

Place the feet in a "V"

Press the shoulders down

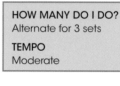

Lengthen the arms back

> **Ready for a challenge?**
> Rise up on the balls of your feet. Lower back down after Step 3.

Standing Side Bends
Focus on flow

Often the simplest moves are the best. To tone the hard-to-reach sides of the body, use Standing Side Bends. As you progress, test your stamina by seeing how long you can sustain the position.

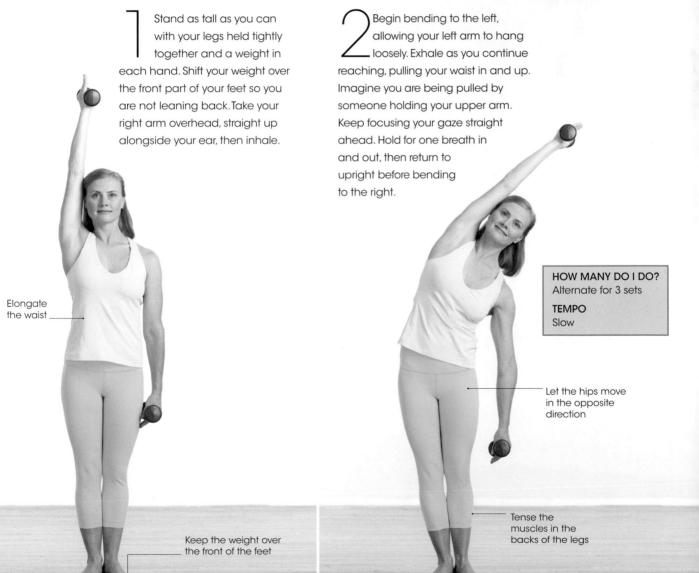

1 Stand as tall as you can with your legs held tightly together and a weight in each hand. Shift your weight over the front part of your feet so you are not leaning back. Take your right arm overhead, straight up alongside your ear, then inhale.

Elongate the waist

Keep the weight over the front of the feet

2 Begin bending to the left, allowing your left arm to hang loosely. Exhale as you continue reaching, pulling your waist in and up. Imagine you are being pulled by someone holding your upper arm. Keep focusing your gaze straight ahead. Hold for one breath in and out, then return to upright before bending to the right.

HOW MANY DO I DO?
Alternate for 3 sets

TEMPO
Slow

Let the hips move in the opposite direction

Tense the muscles in the backs of the legs

15-minute sequence

This basic workout has all the fundamental Pilates moves and principles you need to establish a strong Pilates foundation. Even when you're an advanced practitioner, always come back to your basic workout to strengthen your practice.

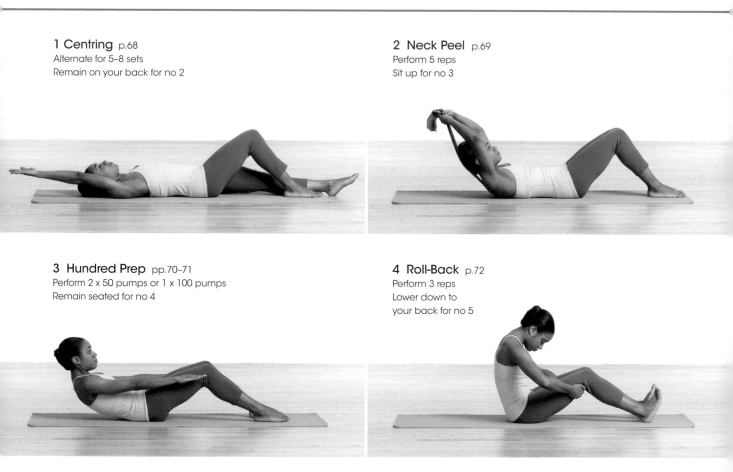

1 Centring p.68
Alternate for 5–8 sets
Remain on your back for no 2

2 Neck Peel p.69
Perform 5 reps
Sit up for no 3

3 Hundred Prep pp.70–71
Perform 2 x 50 pumps or 1 x 100 pumps
Remain seated for no 4

4 Roll-Back p.72
Perform 3 reps
Lower down to
your back for no 5

5 Leg Circles p.74
Perform 5–8 reps, then reverse direction
for 5–8 reps
Flip onto your stomach for no 6

6 Swan Prep p.83
Perform 3–5 reps
Roll onto your left side for no 7

7 Side Kicks: Front I p.85
Perform 8 reps on each side
Come up to standing for no 8

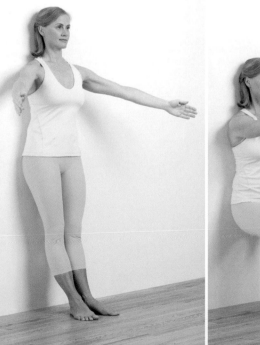

8 Windmill p.92
Perform 3 reps
Stand against a wall
for no 9

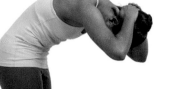

9 Wall: Stand p.96
Stand for 5-10 breaths
Remain at the wall
for no 10

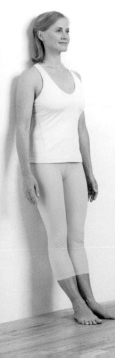

10 Wall: Circles p.97
Perform 3 reps, then reverse
direction for 3 reps
Stay against the wall
for no 11

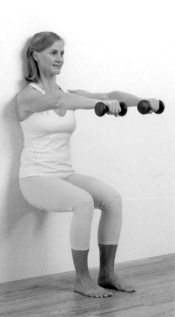

11 Wall: Chair p.98
Perform 2 reps
Step away from the wall
for no 12

**12 Standing
Side Bends** p.103
Alternate for 3 sets

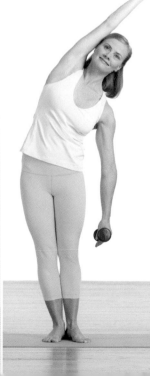

30-minute sequence

A 30-minute workout every day is ideal. But don't let the extra time commitment overwhelm you. Even if you can't set aside a full 30 minutes, you can perform this workout in two separate 15-minute segments.

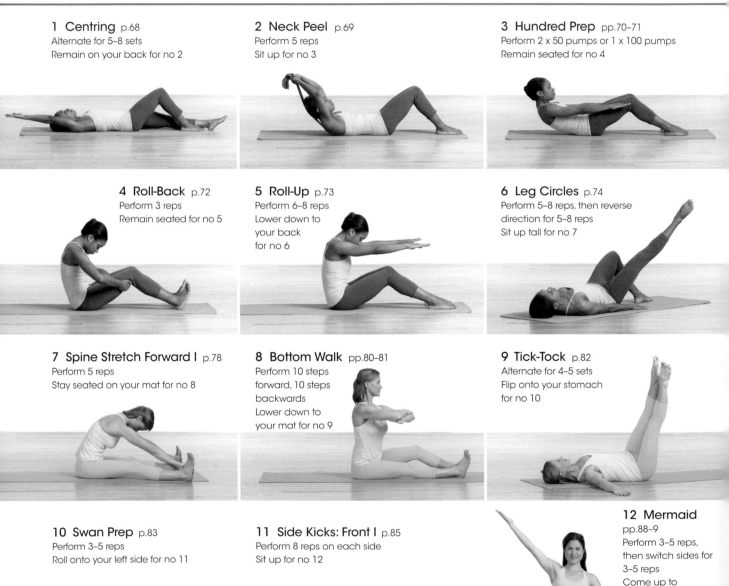

1 Centring p.68
Alternate for 5–8 sets
Remain on your back for no 2

2 Neck Peel p.69
Perform 5 reps
Sit up for no 3

3 Hundred Prep pp.70–71
Perform 2 x 50 pumps or 1 x 100 pumps
Remain seated for no 4

4 Roll-Back p.72
Perform 3 reps
Remain seated for no 5

5 Roll-Up p.73
Perform 6–8 reps
Lower down to your back for no 6

6 Leg Circles p.74
Perform 5–8 reps, then reverse direction for 5–8 reps
Sit up tall for no 7

7 Spine Stretch Forward I p.78
Perform 5 reps
Stay seated on your mat for no 8

8 Bottom Walk pp.80–81
Perform 10 steps forward, 10 steps backwards
Lower down to your mat for no 9

9 Tick-Tock p.82
Alternate for 4–5 sets
Flip onto your stomach for no 10

10 Swan Prep p.83
Perform 3–5 reps
Roll onto your left side for no 11

11 Side Kicks: Front I p.85
Perform 8 reps on each side
Sit up for no 12

12 Mermaid pp.88–9
Perform 3–5 reps, then switch sides for 3–5 reps
Come up to standing for no 13

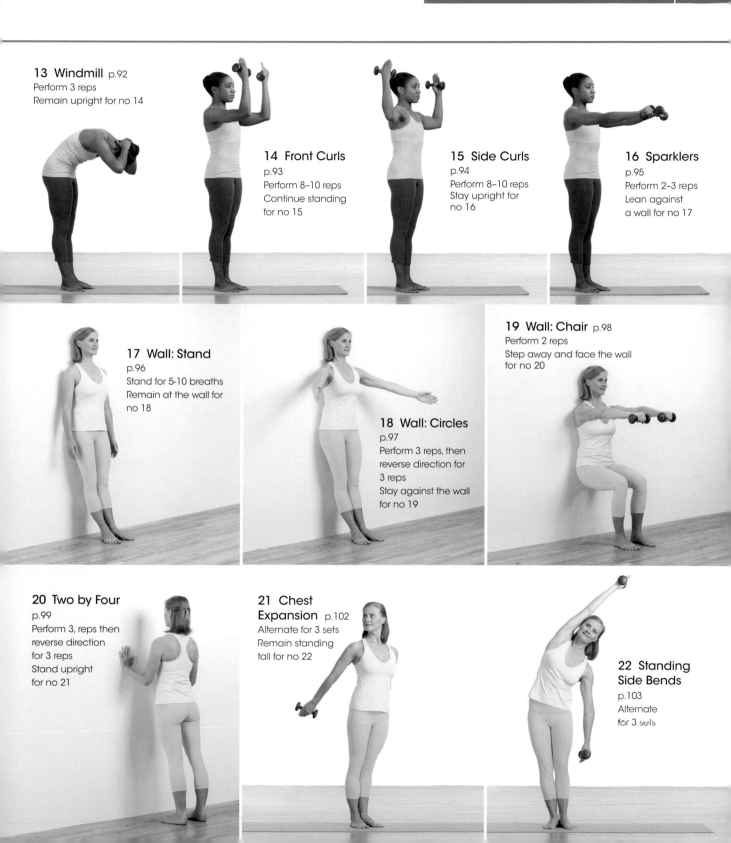

13 Windmill p.92
Perform 3 reps
Remain upright for no 14

14 Front Curls
p.93
Perform 8–10 reps
Continue standing
for no 15

15 Side Curls
p.94
Perform 8–10 reps
Stay upright for
no 16

16 Sparklers
p.95
Perform 2–3 reps
Lean against
a wall for no 17

17 Wall: Stand
p.96
Stand for 5-10 breaths
Remain at the wall for
no 18

18 Wall: Circles
p.97
Perform 3 reps, then
reverse direction for
3 reps
Stay against the wall
for no 19

19 Wall: Chair p.98
Perform 2 reps
Step away and face the wall
for no 20

20 Two by Four
p.99
Perform 3, reps then
reverse direction
for 3 reps
Stand upright
for no 21

**21 Chest
Expansion** p.102
Alternate for 3 sets
Remain standing
tall for no 22

**22 Standing
Side Bends**
p.103
Alternate
for 3 sets

45-minute sequence

If you have the luxury of being able to devote 45 minutes to your workout, then dive into this programme. The moves are more complex than you've been used to so far and the order of movements has changed now that you're getting better and better.

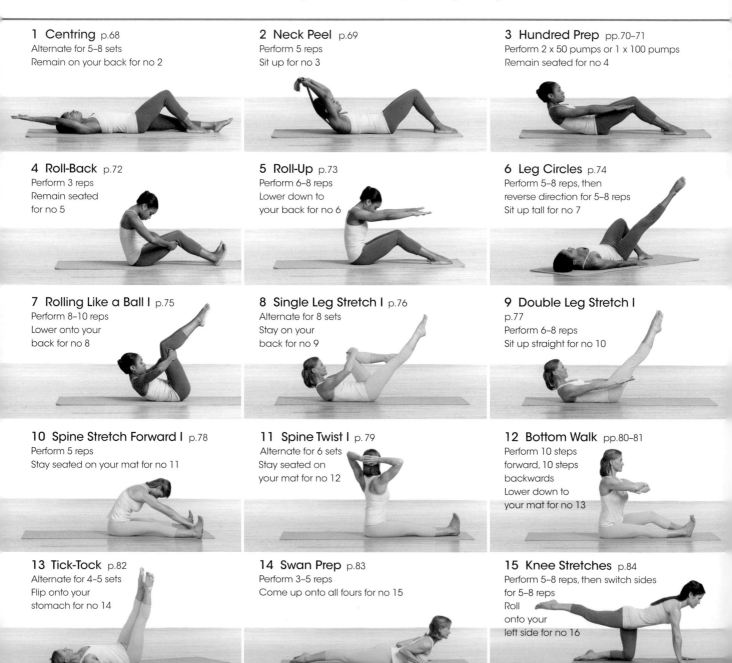

1 Centring p.68
Alternate for 5–8 sets
Remain on your back for no 2

2 Neck Peel p.69
Perform 5 reps
Sit up for no 3

3 Hundred Prep pp.70–71
Perform 2 x 50 pumps or 1 x 100 pumps
Remain seated for no 4

4 Roll-Back p.72
Perform 3 reps
Remain seated
for no 5

5 Roll-Up p.73
Perform 6–8 reps
Lower down to
your back for no 6

6 Leg Circles p.74
Perform 5–8 reps, then
reverse direction for 5–8 reps
Sit up tall for no 7

7 Rolling Like a Ball I p.75
Perform 8–10 reps
Lower onto your
back for no 8

8 Single Leg Stretch I p.76
Alternate for 8 sets
Stay on your
back for no 9

9 Double Leg Stretch I
p.77
Perform 6–8 reps
Sit up straight for no 10

10 Spine Stretch Forward I p.78
Perform 5 reps
Stay seated on your mat for no 11

11 Spine Twist I p.79
Alternate for 6 sets
Stay seated on
your mat for no 12

12 Bottom Walk pp.80–81
Perform 10 steps
forward, 10 steps
backwards
Lower down to
your mat for no 13

13 Tick-Tock p.82
Alternate for 4–5 sets
Flip onto your
stomach for no 14

14 Swan Prep p.83
Perform 3–5 reps
Come up onto all fours for no 15

15 Knee Stretches p.84
Perform 5–8 reps, then switch sides
for 5–8 reps
Roll
onto your
left side for no 16

16 Side Kicks: Front I p.85
Perform 8 reps
Stay on your side for no 17

17 Side Kicks: Double Leg Lift p.86
Perform 5 reps
Remain on your side for no 18

18 Side Kicks: Lower Lift p.87
Perform 8 reps, then switch sides and repeat
numbers 16, 17 and 18 on your right side
Sit up tall for no 19

19 Mermaid
pp.88–9
Perform 3–5 reps,
then switch sides for
3–5 reps
Lie back on your
mat for no 20

20 Shoulder Bridge p.90–91
Perform 5 reps, then switch sides for 5 reps
Come up to standing for no 21

21 Windmill
p.92
Perform 3 reps
Come up to
standing for no 22

22 Front Curls p.93
Perform 8–10 reps
Stay upright for no 23

23 Side Curls p.94
Perform 8–10 reps
Continue standing for
no 24

24 Sparklers p.95
Perform 2–3 reps
Lean against a wall for
no 25

25 Wall: Stand p.96
Stand for 5-10 breaths
Remain at the wall for
no 26

26 Wall: Circles p.97
Perform 3 reps, then reverse
direction for 3 reps
Remain at the wall for no 27

27 Wall: Chair
p.98
Perform 2 reps
Step away and face
the wall for no 28

28 Two by Four p.99
Perform 3 reps, then reverse
direction for 3 reps
Come into a
lunge for no 29

29 Front Splits
pp.100–101
Perform 1 full set on
each side
Stand up tall for no 30

30 Chest Expansion
p.102
Alternate for 3 sets
Stay upright for no 31

**31 Standing Side
Bends** p.103
Alternate
for 3 sets

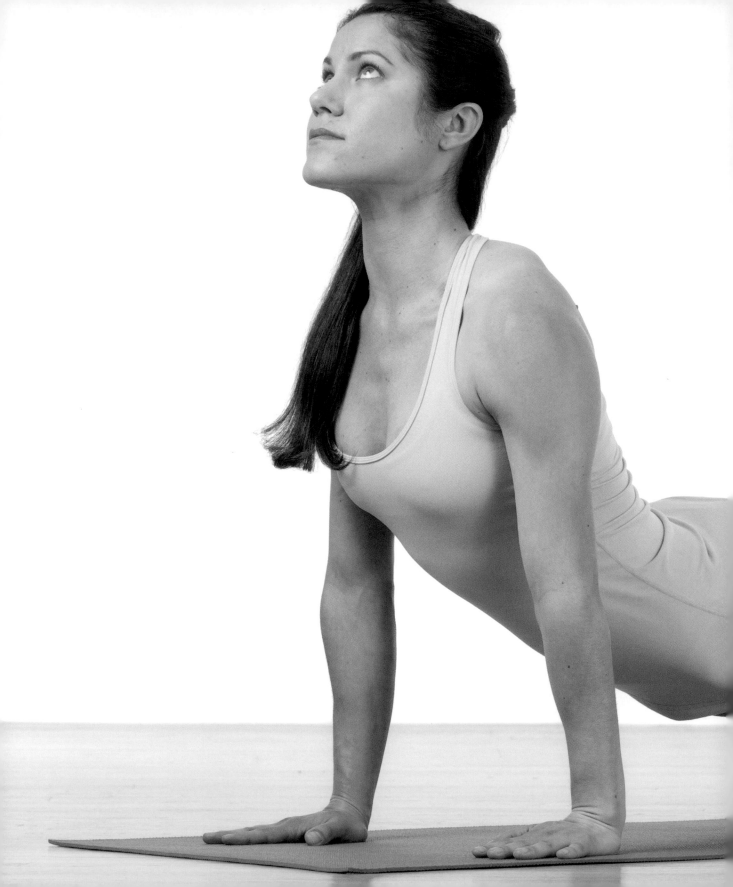

Intermediate

Get ready to take your training to the next level with the Intermediate programme. These moves will add new ingredients to the mix. Keep all your Beginner moves in your mind as you tackle this new programme.

Ten by Ten
Focus on breath

The classic Pilates Hundred exercise can be done a dozen different ways – and this is one of them. As you begin your Intermediate programme, your goals for this exercise will be to build stamina, increase your abdominal strength and control, and to warm up.

1 Start sitting up towards the front of your mat with your knees bent and pressed together. Stretch your arms straight ahead, fire up your abs (see p.57) and begin lowering yourself slowly backwards to the mat. Let your hips round under you so you can really curl through your lower back.

2 Continue lowering until the base of your shoulders reaches the floor. You should be in a good abdominal crunch, with your arms parallel with and extended above your thighs. Extend your right leg, keeping your inner thighs pressed together.

Scoop the abs strongly

Work the inner thigh muscles together

3 Now extend your left leg to meet your right leg. Keep stretching your arms forward, then bounce your arms up and down in a pumping motion. Breathe in for 5 pumps, then out for 5 pumps, then hold still for 1 full inhalation and 1 full exhalation. Repeat the pumping and breathing cycles until you have performed 100 pumps.

HOW MANY DO I DO?
Perform 100 pumps

TEMPO
Rapid

Keep the feet together

Breathe out through the mouth

Use the abs to hold the head up

Pump the arms above the torso

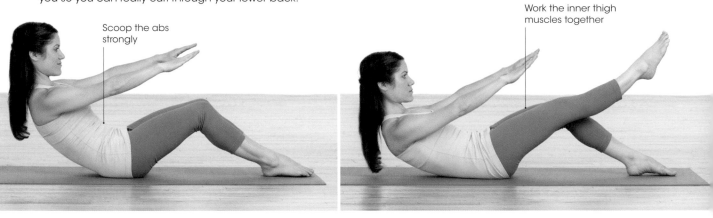

Half Roll-Up
Focus on control

Roll-Up is the perfect exercise to build strength and articulate the spine. This truncated version will force you to use your abdominals properly and eliminate the tendency to lurch up or substitute other muscles for the abs.

1 Sit up with your upper body rounded over your legs. Stretch your arms over your legs, flex your feet and keep your head low. Scoop your abs in (see p.61).

2 Inhale, then pull yourself back down towards the mat until you are at the lowest and most challenging portion of the descent for your level of strength. Now freeze. Hold for 3 full breaths.

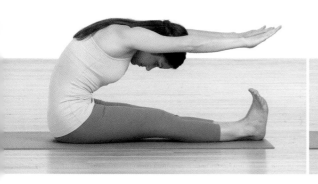

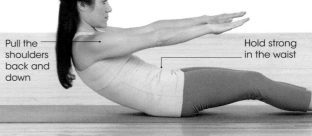

Pull the shoulders back and down

Hold strong in the waist

3 Pull your abs in even tighter. Tense your leg muscles and exhale fully as you round back up to where you began. With each repetition, hold a bit longer and challenge yourself to go just a bit lower.

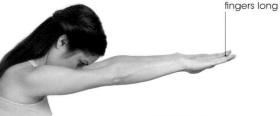

Keep the fingers long

HOW MANY DO I DO?
Perform 5 reps

TEMPO
Slow

Resist rounding forward

Work the glutes

Mini Bridge
Focus on concentration

Mini Bridge is not part of the traditional repertoire but it is essential for strength-building. This simple motion and single-plane movement leaves no stone unturned. It targets the back, or posterior, muscles from the legs to the back, and even the arms.

1 Lie flat on your mat in a straight line. Align your legs with the centre of the mat and flex your feet. Press your arms and palms into the mat underneath you. Breathe naturally.

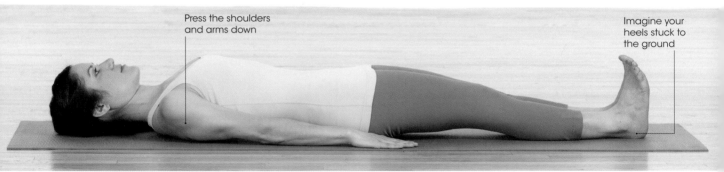

Press the shoulders and arms down

Imagine your heels stuck to the ground

2 In one motion and propelling yourself from your hips, lift your bottom up off the mat. Balance on your shoulders, hands and heels. Keep your legs, including your heels and toes, pulling in towards each other along their entire length. Imagine you are eliminating all the space between your legs. Hold for 5 full breaths. Lower and pause before repeating.

HOW MANY DO I DO?
Perform 3 reps

TEMPO
Slow

Keep the ribs in

Use the hips to power you up

Point the knees and feet straight up

Rolling Like a Ball II
Focus on precision

You prepared for Rolling Like a Ball in the Beginner programme (see p.75). This is the next progression. Don't expect to master it quickly. Use patience and persistence. Over time you will develop a balance of strength and control as well as momentum.

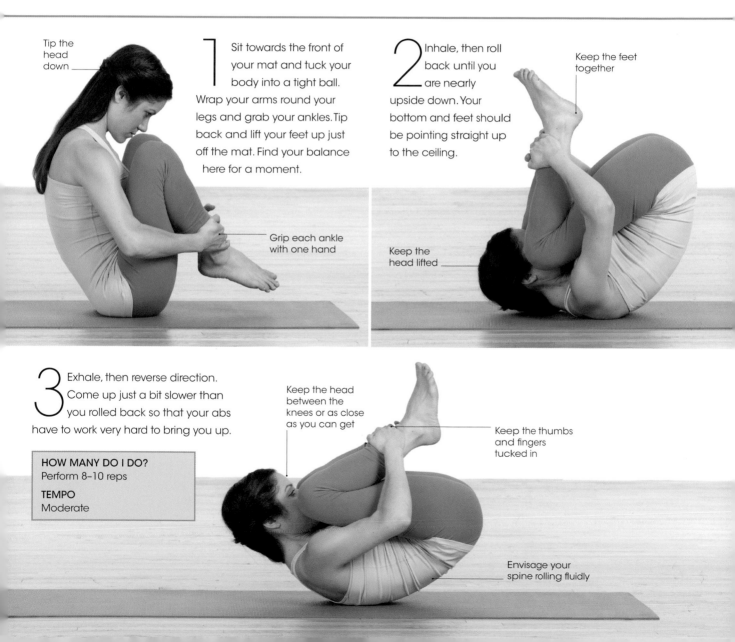

Tip the head down

1 Sit towards the front of your mat and tuck your body into a tight ball. Wrap your arms round your legs and grab your ankles. Tip back and lift your feet up just off the mat. Find your balance here for a moment.

Grip each ankle with one hand

2 Inhale, then roll back until you are nearly upside down. Your bottom and feet should be pointing straight up to the ceiling.

Keep the feet together

Keep the head lifted

3 Exhale, then reverse direction. Come up just a bit slower than you rolled back so that your abs have to work very hard to bring you up.

Keep the head between the knees or as close as you can get

Keep the thumbs and fingers tucked in

Envisage your spine rolling fluidly

HOW MANY DO I DO?
Perform 8–10 reps

TEMPO
Moderate

Coordination
Focus on concentration

In this programme we borrow several exercises from the Pilates Reformer machine (see p.217). Although you don't work with springs in the mat work, you should work with resistance as though the springs were there. Coordination helps you practise this.

1 Lie on your back with your knees into your chest. Use your abs to lift your head, neck and shoulders off the mat. Press your elbows into the mat and bend your forearms to vertical.

Hug the sides of the body with the arms

2 Inhale and extend your arms and legs forward without losing control of your abs or lowering your head. Take your arms to the mat and hold your legs at the lowest point you can support while keeping your torso solid. Try to curl your upper body higher the whole time.

Lengthen the legs away from the torso

Relax the neck and shoulders

Keep the palms flat on the floor

3 Hold for a second as you open your legs just past hip-width. Use resistance as though you were trying to push your legs apart against something heavy. Now bring your legs back together with the same resistance, pulling your abs in once again.

Open and close the legs with resistance

Work the abs

4 Exhale deeply as you bend your knees tightly into your chest. Keep exhaling as you bend your forearms back into their vertical, Step 1 position.

HOW MANY DO I DO?
Perform 5 reps

TEMPO
Moderate

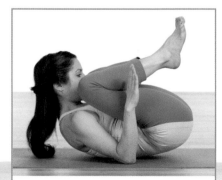

Ready for a challenge?
Try pulling your knees in so tightly to your body that your hips curl up slightly off the mat.

Lift the shoulders higher to bend the legs in

Single Leg Stretch II
Focus on precision

This variation of Single Leg Stretch I (see p.76) addresses your coordination and timing, so it is critical that you keep an internal dialogue going. Say the words in your mind as your body makes the motions. Assigning words to movements develops muscle memory.

1 Lie flat, then curl up high as you hug your right leg into your chest. Place your right hand on your right ankle and your left hand on your knee. Stretch your left leg out on a high diagonal down the midline of your body (see p.57). Squeeze your glutes and inhale to begin.

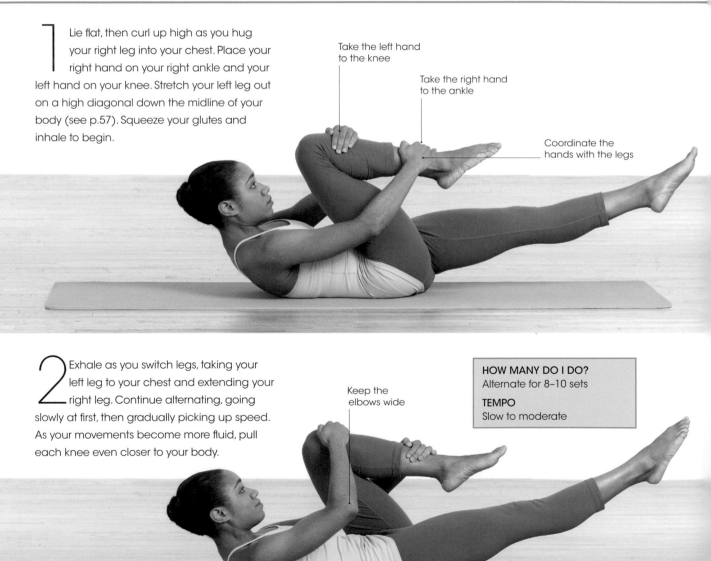

Take the left hand to the knee

Take the right hand to the ankle

Coordinate the hands with the legs

2 Exhale as you switch legs, taking your left leg to your chest and extending your right leg. Continue alternating, going slowly at first, then gradually picking up speed. As your movements become more fluid, pull each knee even closer to your body.

Keep the elbows wide

Hold strong in the torso

Maintain tight glutes

HOW MANY DO I DO?
Alternate for 8–10 sets

TEMPO
Slow to moderate

Double Leg Stretch II

Focus on breath

Recall the Centring exercise (see p.68) where you learned to initiate from the core and lengthen your limbs fully. Double Leg Stretch II will reinforce those habits. You've met this exercise before in the Beginner programme (see p.77), but this version goes further.

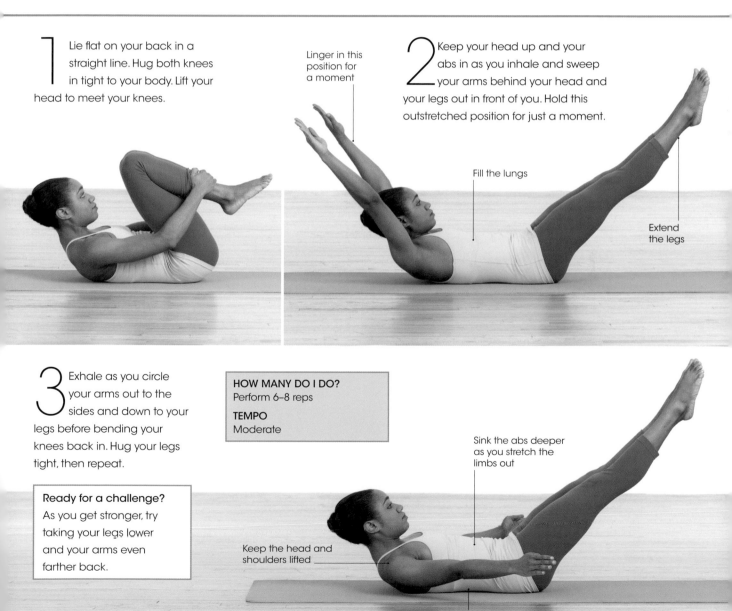

1 Lie flat on your back in a straight line. Hug both knees in tight to your body. Lift your head to meet your knees.

2 Keep your head up and your abs in as you inhale and sweep your arms behind your head and your legs out in front of you. Hold this outstretched position for just a moment.

Linger in this position for a moment

Fill the lungs

Extend the legs

3 Exhale as you circle your arms out to the sides and down to your legs before bending your knees back in. Hug your legs tight, then repeat.

HOW MANY DO I DO?
Perform 6–8 reps

TEMPO
Moderate

Sink the abs deeper as you stretch the limbs out

Ready for a challenge?
As you get stronger, try taking your legs lower and your arms even farther back.

Keep the head and shoulders lifted

Keep the back flat

Single Straight Leg Stretch
Focus on flow

Instructors often refer to this exercise by the name "Scissors", which reflects the brisk, sharp action of the legs. This up-tempo move demonstrates how a solid core can allow the limbs to move at lightning speed with no strain to the torso.

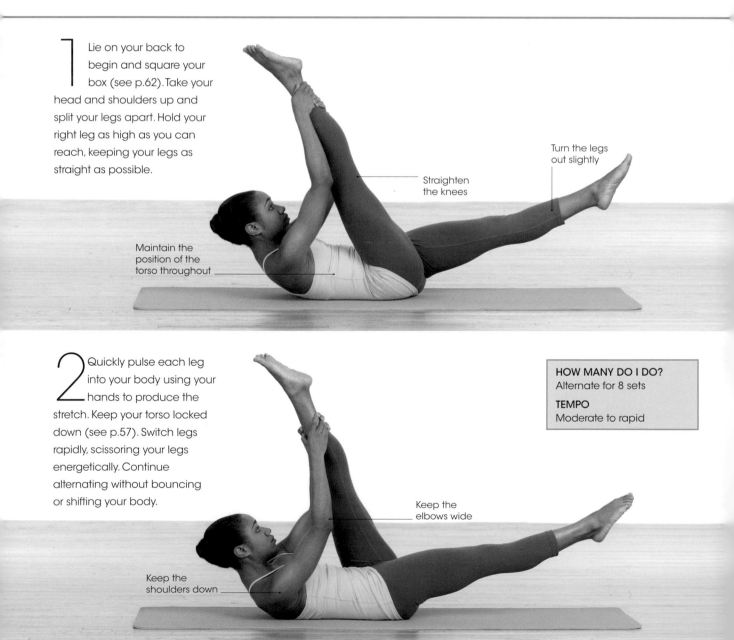

1 Lie on your back to begin and square your box (see p.62). Take your head and shoulders up and split your legs apart. Hold your right leg as high as you can reach, keeping your legs as straight as possible.

Straighten the knees

Turn the legs out slightly

Maintain the position of the torso throughout

2 Quickly pulse each leg into your body using your hands to produce the stretch. Keep your torso locked down (see p.57). Switch legs rapidly, scissoring your legs energetically. Continue alternating without bouncing or shifting your body.

HOW MANY DO I DO?
Alternate for 8 sets

TEMPO
Moderate to rapid

Keep the elbows wide

Keep the shoulders down

Spine Stretch Forward II
Focus on centring

Spine Stretch Forward changes as you advance in your Pilates. Work on your C-curve (see p.63), this time with a long, lifted waist and high arms. Avoid any shrinking or compressing. Instead, create your letter "C" by lengthening the spine and then curving it up even higher.

1 Sit upright with your legs straight ahead and just wider than your hips. Make sure your legs are facing straight up to the ceiling. Flex your feet. Raise your arms overhead and inhale.

Keep the knees facing the ceiling

2 Lift up very high and very tall, then round forward as you begin a slow, deep exhalation. Keep your arms in line with your ears as you come into your C-curve. Imagine someone is pulling you forward by your fingertips as you resist. Keep working the muscles of your legs.

Empty the lungs

Maintain tight buttock muscles

3 From your deepest C-curve, inhale and roll up again to bring your upper body back to your starting position. Press your shoulders down and lengthen your neck. Do not relax your waist or your legs. Stay poised for the next repetition.

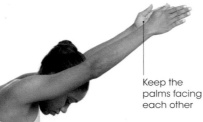

Keep the palms facing each other

Hollow out the abs

HOW MANY DO I DO?
Perform 5 reps

TEMPO
Slow

Corkscrew
Focus on precision

Pilates alternates between exercises that focus on a single concept and moves that challenge many elements all at once. Corkscrew challenges all of your abdominals simultaneously. The rectus abdominis, obliques and transversus must all go to work.

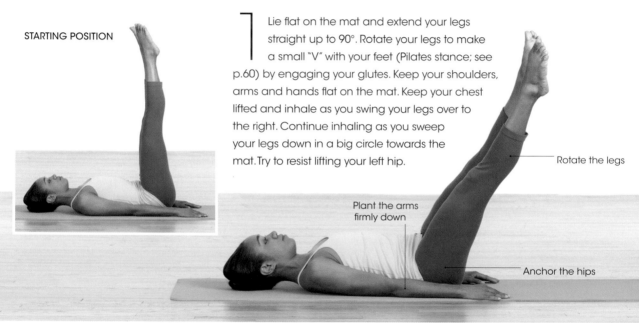

STARTING POSITION

1 Lie flat on the mat and extend your legs straight up to 90°. Rotate your legs to make a small "V" with your feet (Pilates stance; see p.60) by engaging your glutes. Keep your shoulders, arms and hands flat on the mat. Keep your chest lifted and inhale as you swing your legs over to the right. Continue inhaling as you sweep your legs down in a big circle towards the mat. Try to resist lifting your left hip.

Rotate the legs

Plant the arms firmly down

Anchor the hips

2 Once you reach the lowest point of the circle, start to exhale as you circle your legs up to the left. Circle back up to your starting point with your legs at a 90° angle. Repeat, this time swinging your legs in a big circle to the left.

HOW MANY DO I DO?
Alternate for 5 sets

TEMPO
Moderate

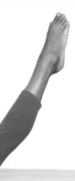

Keep the shoulders down

Letter T
Focus on breath

Hand weights are optional for this move, which develops the muscles in the upper back to help you stand tall and healthy. Keep the focus in the upper back as you practise this move, to avoid straining your lower-back muscles.

1 Lie face-down on your stomach with your legs together. Lift your head and chest slightly and stretch your arms out to the sides of the room. You may hold a hand weight in each hand. Keep your palms facing the floor.

Lock down the legs

Lift the abs

Keep the palms face down

2 Exhale as you sweep your arms smoothly back behind you, lifting your chin and chest, but leaving your waist on the mat. Think of opening your chest forward rather than lifting higher. Work the muscles in your upper back to retract your shoulders and bring your arms closer to your body. Inhale as you release with control to return to the starting position.

HOW MANY DO I DO?
Perform 5 reps

TEMPO
Slow

Reach the arms higher than the body

Linger at the highest point of the lift

Keep the feet pressed into the floor

Keep the legs on the mat

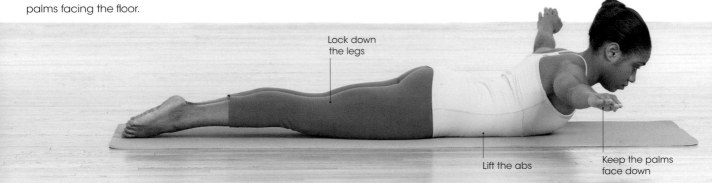

Round Back
Focus on concentration

Your body learns from visual, verbal and tactile cues. Tactile cues are the strongest cues you can give your muscles. In this exercise, use the pressure of your arms to train your tummy muscles to contract deeper with each repetition.

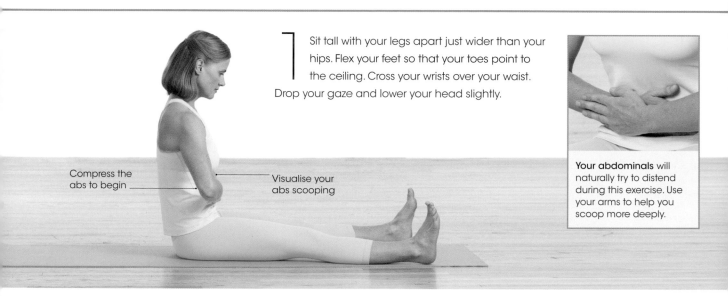

1 Sit tall with your legs apart just wider than your hips. Flex your feet so that your toes point to the ceiling. Cross your wrists over your waist. Drop your gaze and lower your head slightly.

Compress the abs to begin

Visualise your abs scooping

Your abdominals will naturally try to distend during this exercise. Use your arms to help you scoop more deeply.

2 Inhale as you round back, pressing into your abs with your arms. The farther back you go, the greater the pressure on your abs should be. Curl to your lowest possible point. Pause here for 3 breaths, pulling your navel towards your spine. Keep working your leg muscles strongly.

Curl the pelvis under as you lower

Firm the legs

Stretch the lower back

3 Exhale and begin to round back up. Continue to pull your navel towards your spine and keep pressing your forearms into your abs. Round back over your legs and begin once again.

Press the shoulders down

HOW MANY DO I DO?
Perform 5 reps

TEMPO
Moderate

Push the heels forward with resistance

Flat Back

Focus on control

Muscles only know how to contract, or shorten. Whether you activate them in a shortened or lengthened position, they will still contract. Flat Back requires a muscle contraction during lengthening (see pp.30–31). This is known as an eccentric contraction.

1 Sit tall with your legs just beyond hip-width. Stretch your arms overhead, holding a band or weighted bar (see p.52) between your hands, or simply hook your thumbs together. Press your shoulders down by using the muscles under your shoulder blades to pull together towards the centre of your back. Pull the band taut to begin.

2 Look straight ahead. Squeeze your buttock muscles, then inhale and lean back, taking your arms with you and tightening your abs the whole time. Go to your lowest point. Pause for a breath, then exhale to return upright.

HOW MANY DO I DO?
Perform 5 reps

TEMPO
Slow

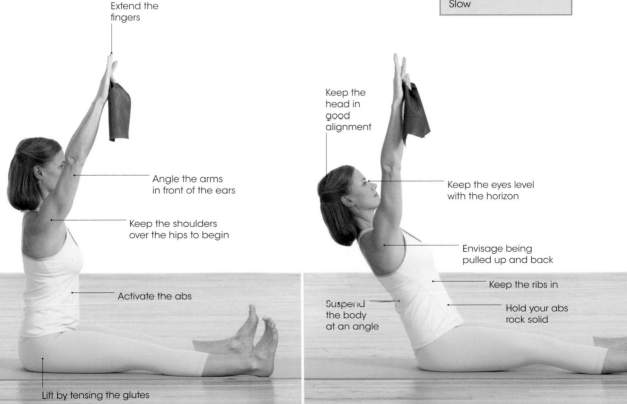

Extend the fingers

Angle the arms in front of the ears

Keep the shoulders over the hips to begin

Activate the abs

Lift by tensing the glutes

Keep the head in good alignment

Keep the eyes level with the horizon

Envisage being pulled up and back

Keep the ribs in

Suspend the body at an angle

Hold your abs rock solid

Side to Side
Focus on precision

Lateral movements help us to work with opposition. As you stretch and bend in Side to Side, notice how your lower body must stabilise and anchor as your upper body extends away. Carry this concept and feeling into other exercises.

1 Sit tall with your legs just beyond hip-width and bring your arms overhead, holding a band or weighted bar. Alternatively, you can hook your thumbs together. Inhale as you tense your leg muscles and flex your feet. Tighten your glutes to begin.

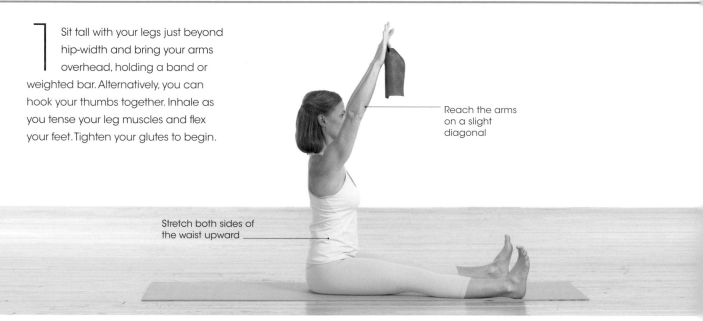

Reach the arms on a slight diagonal

Stretch both sides of the waist upward

2 Sit even taller, then exhale as you bend to the right. Resist with your left hip, creating a strong stretch in your left side. Reach up and out, not down. At your farthest point, pause for a moment. Exhale and reach out a little farther, then spring back up to the centre. Inhale to prepare, then exhale to repeat on the other side.

HOW MANY DO I DO?
Alternate for 3 sets

TEMPO
Moderate

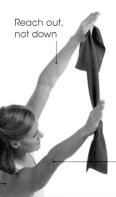

Reach out, not down

Keep stretching the bottom arm

Reach very slightly forward

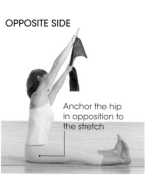

OPPOSITE SIDE

Anchor the hip in opposition to the stretch

Twist and Reach
Focus on centring

Pilates promises to whittle the waist. Twist and Reach accomplishes this feat nicely by strengthening and toning the obliques. Weak obliques are believed to contribute to the appearance of "love handles", so don't skip this one.

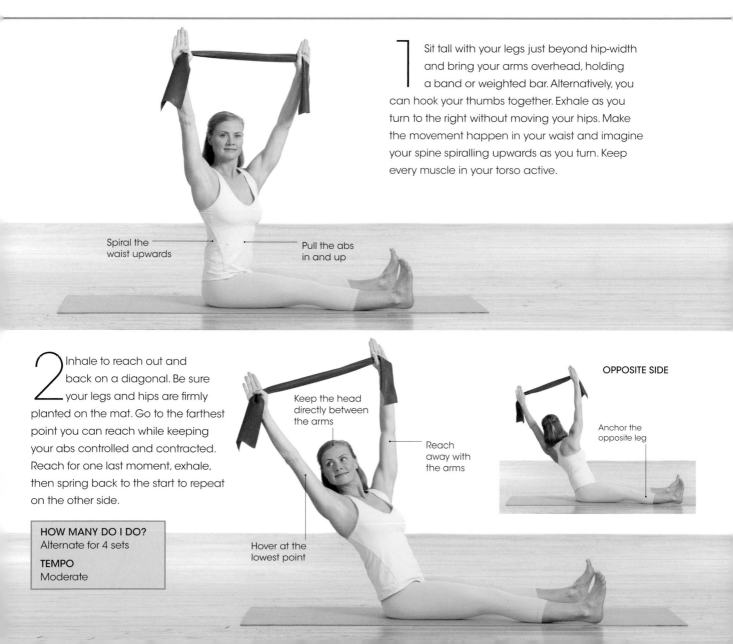

1 Sit tall with your legs just beyond hip-width and bring your arms overhead, holding a band or weighted bar. Alternatively, you can hook your thumbs together. Exhale as you turn to the right without moving your hips. Make the movement happen in your waist and imagine your spine spiralling upwards as you turn. Keep every muscle in your torso active.

Spiral the waist upwards

Pull the abs in and up

2 Inhale to reach out and back on a diagonal. Be sure your legs and hips are firmly planted on the mat. Go to the farthest point you can reach while keeping your abs controlled and contracted. Reach for one last moment, exhale, then spring back to the start to repeat on the other side.

HOW MANY DO I DO?
Alternate for 4 sets

TEMPO
Moderate

Keep the head directly between the arms

Reach away with the arms

Hover at the lowest point

OPPOSITE SIDE

Anchor the opposite leg

Neck Pull
Focus on control

Exercise is simply physics. By repositioning legs, arms or weights, we can make dramatic changes in how much we load a muscle. This is a challenging exercise. It makes greater demands on the abdominals by having the arms behind the head.

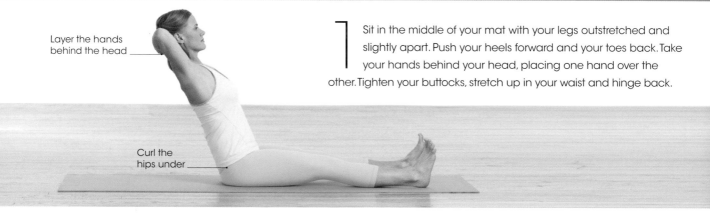

Layer the hands behind the head

Curl the hips under

1 Sit in the middle of your mat with your legs outstretched and slightly apart. Push your heels forward and your toes back. Take your hands behind your head, placing one hand over the other. Tighten your buttocks, stretch up in your waist and hinge back.

Keep the elbows wide

Scoop the abs

2 Inhale as you go to the lowest point you can while still keeping your waist pulled in and your spine straight and long. When you cannot go any farther, bring your head forward, curl your hips under and begin to exhale.

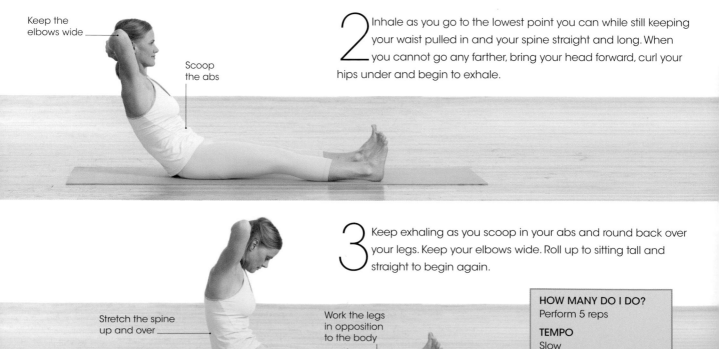

3 Keep exhaling as you scoop in your abs and round back over your legs. Keep your elbows wide. Roll up to sitting tall and straight to begin again.

Stretch the spine up and over

Work the legs in opposition to the body

HOW MANY DO I DO?
Perform 5 reps

TEMPO
Slow

Semicircle
Focus on concentration

As your Pilates practice improves, the positions and choreography become more complex. Created for the Pilates Reformer machine, this adapted exercise blends spinal articulation with hip strength and mobility.

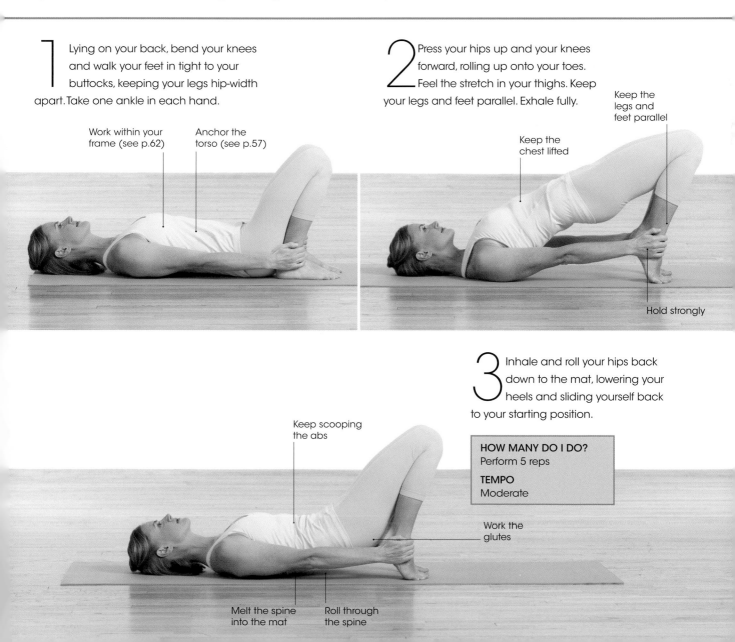

1 Lying on your back, bend your knees and walk your feet in tight to your buttocks, keeping your legs hip-width apart. Take one ankle in each hand.

Work within your frame (see p.62)

Anchor the torso (see p.57)

2 Press your hips up and your knees forward, rolling up onto your toes. Feel the stretch in your thighs. Keep your legs and feet parallel. Exhale fully.

Keep the legs and feet parallel

Keep the chest lifted

Hold strongly

3 Inhale and roll your hips back down to the mat, lowering your heels and sliding yourself back to your starting position.

Keep scooping the abs

HOW MANY DO I DO?
Perform 5 reps

TEMPO
Moderate

Work the glutes

Melt the spine into the mat

Roll through the spine

Side Kicks: Front II
Focus on centring

As in the Beginner programme, perform all the Side Kicks Series (pp.130–33) to one side before switching to the other leg. Tiny adjustments can completely change an exercise, as you'll see from the changes made to this version.

1 Lie on your left side with your hips and shoulders lined up at the back edge of the mat. Place your head on your left hand and your right hand behind your head. Take your legs forward to the front edge of your mat. Keep your legs parallel. Inhale to begin.

Stack the hips and shoulders in one line

2 Lift your right leg and exhale as you kick to the front with a double pulse. Resist any rounding in your lower back or tucking under in your pelvis. Keep your chest lifted and your abs tight.

Keep the knee straight

Plant the bottom leg firmly

3 Exhale as you sweep your right leg as far back as possible while holding it straight. Keep your upper body stable and strong.

Keep the leg at hip height

Hold your box square

Flex the bottom foot

HOW MANY DO I DO?
Perform 10 kicks front and back. Repeat on each side.

TEMPO
Moderate to rapid

Side Kicks: Scissors
Focus on flow

This variation of Side Kicks is not often taught, but I'm including it in this programme to surprise your body and shock your muscles quickly and effectively into activation. This is a move in which you can let loose a little and trust your muscles to do their job.

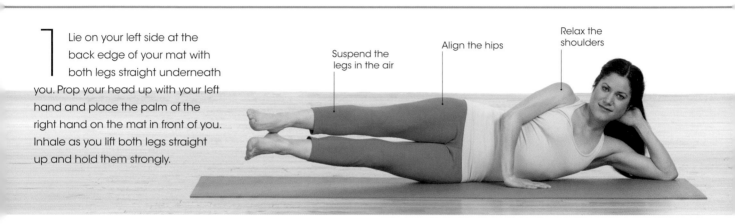

1 Lie on your left side at the back edge of your mat with both legs straight underneath you. Prop your head up with your left hand and place the palm of the right hand on the mat in front of you. Inhale as you lift both legs straight up and hold them strongly.

Suspend the legs in the air

Align the hips

Relax the shoulders

2 Exhale and begin to scissor your legs, carrying your left leg to the front first. Breathe naturally as you begin slowly scissoring your legs back and forth for 6 kicks. Keep your abs strong.

Keep the arches of the feet long

Anchor the torso

3 Gradually pick up speed for 6 more kicks. Do a final 6 kicks until your legs are moving as fast as possible.

Keep the legs straight

HOW MANY DO I DO?
Perform 18 kicks back and forth. Repeat on each side.

TEMPO
Rapid

Side Kicks: Circles
Focus on control

Who needs weights if you know how to get gravity on your side? Flipping onto one side means that we can use gravity for our resistance. Resistance, in turn, creates strength, tone and greater mobility.

1 Lie on your left side with your hips and shoulders lined up at the back edge of the mat. Prop your head up with your left hand and place the palm of the right hand on the mat in front of you. Take your legs forward to the front edge of your mat. Keep your legs parallel. Lift your right leg and take it forward slightly in front of your left leg.

Relax the upper body

Keep the legs long and straight

2 Breathe naturally as you make small deliberate circles with your right foot just in front of your left ankle. As you circle, emphasise the downward movement. Circle 10 times.

Hold the leg at hip level

Lift the underside of the waist

3 Continuing to breathe naturally, switch directions by taking your right leg behind your left leg. Circle once again, this time circling to the back.

Maintain the buttocks at the back edge of the mat

HOW MANY DO I DO?
Perform 10 circles in each direction. Repeat on each side.

TEMPO
Rapid

Side Kicks: Inner Thighs
Focus on precision

Inner thighs are a trouble spot for many exercisers. We tend to neglect those muscles through poor standing and sitting posture, so they are often weak. When you have finished this last exercise in the Side Kicks Series, repeat from p.130 on your right side.

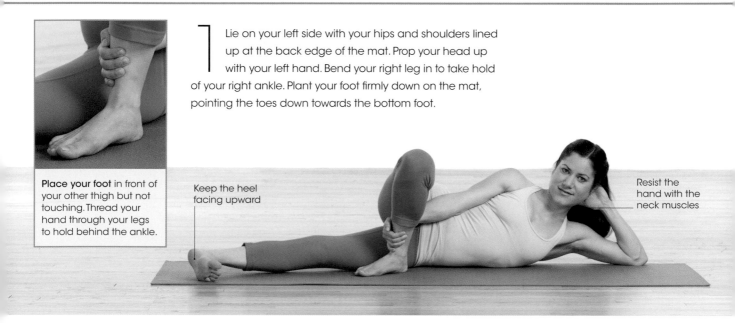

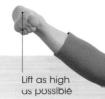

Place your foot in front of your other thigh but not touching. Thread your hand through your legs to hold behind the ankle.

1 Lie on your left side with your hips and shoulders lined up at the back edge of the mat. Prop your head up with your left hand. Bend your right leg in to take hold of your right ankle. Plant your foot firmly down on the mat, pointing the toes down towards the bottom foot.

Keep the heel facing upward

Resist the hand with the neck muscles

2 Draw your abs in tightly as you lift your leg up high, flexing your foot. Emphasise the upward movement. Breathe naturally as you lower and lift your left leg, keeping space between your legs.

HOW MANY DO I DO?
Perform 10 kicks.
Repeat on each side.

TEMPO
Moderate

Keep the eyes looking straight ahead

Keep space between the legs

Lift as high as possible

Relax the bottom shoulder

Backward Teaser
Focus on control

For many people, the Teaser exercise is a source of frustration. By tackling it from a seated position, I've found that almost everyone can do it. Build your strength by starting small and increasing your range of motion more and more each time.

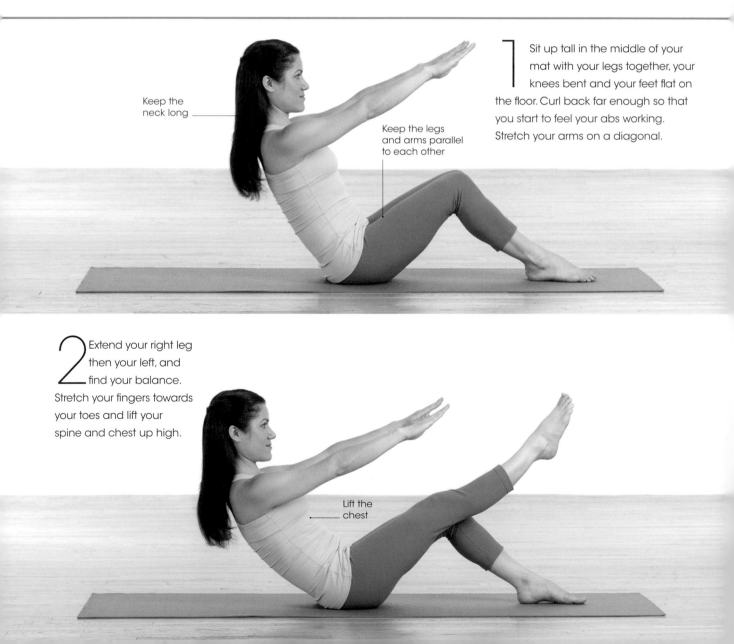

Keep the neck long

Keep the legs and arms parallel to each other

1 Sit up tall in the middle of your mat with your legs together, your knees bent and your feet flat on the floor. Curl back far enough so that you start to feel your abs working. Stretch your arms on a diagonal.

2 Extend your right leg then your left, and find your balance. Stretch your fingers towards your toes and lift your spine and chest up high.

Lift the chest

3 Inhale and curl down smoothly, lowering your back towards the mat. Keep your legs stable and strong. Avoid the urge to let your abdominals distend.

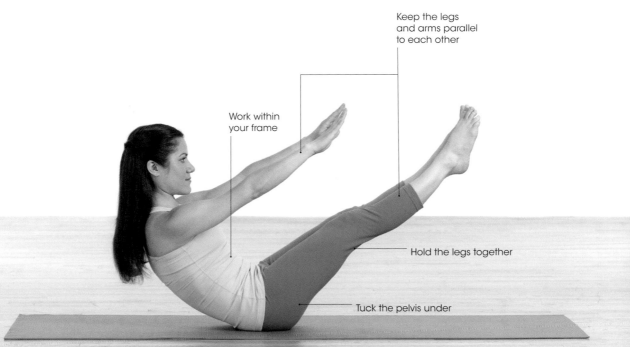

Keep the legs and arms parallel to each other

Work within your frame

Hold the legs together

Tuck the pelvis under

4 Exhale and rise back up, making a perfect letter "V" with your spine and legs. Continue lowering down and rising up, going progressively lower with each repetition. Bend your knees and sit up tall to finish.

HOW MANY DO I DO?
Perform 4–6 reps

TEMPO
Slow

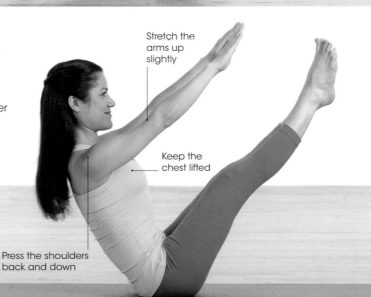

Stretch the arms up slightly

Keep the chest lifted

Press the shoulders back and down

Teaser with Twist
Focus on centring

Often seen as a preparatory version, I consider this version of the classic Teaser exercise to be far more challenging. Here you'll be working your obliques as well as your rectus abdominis, which will double the workload on your muscles.

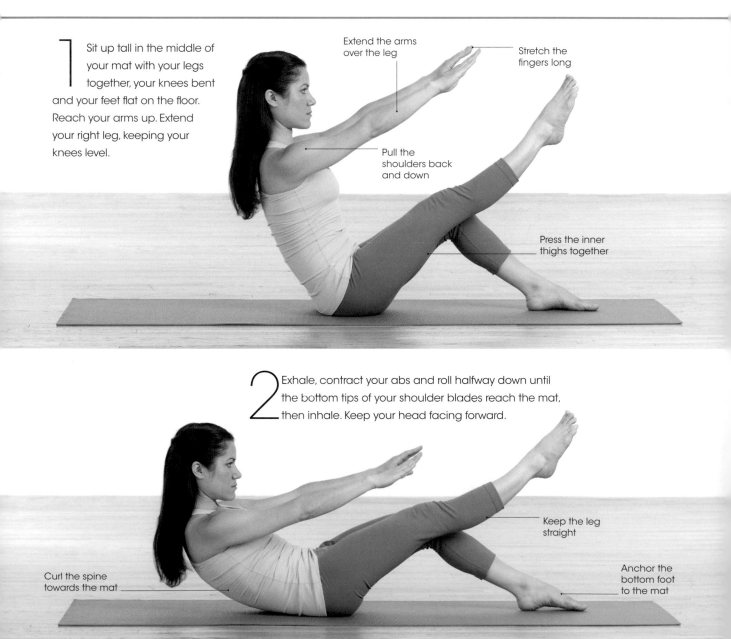

1 Sit up tall in the middle of your mat with your legs together, your knees bent and your feet flat on the floor. Reach your arms up. Extend your right leg, keeping your knees level.

Extend the arms over the leg

Stretch the fingers long

Pull the shoulders back and down

Press the inner thighs together

2 Exhale, contract your abs and roll halfway down until the bottom tips of your shoulder blades reach the mat, then inhale. Keep your head facing forward.

Keep the leg straight

Curl the spine towards the mat

Anchor the bottom foot to the mat

3 Exhale again and curl back up, then twist your body over your extended right leg. Keep your back long and your abs in and up. Return to the centre to lower once again.

HOW MANY DO I DO?
Perform 3 reps, then switch sides for 3 reps
TEMPO
Moderate

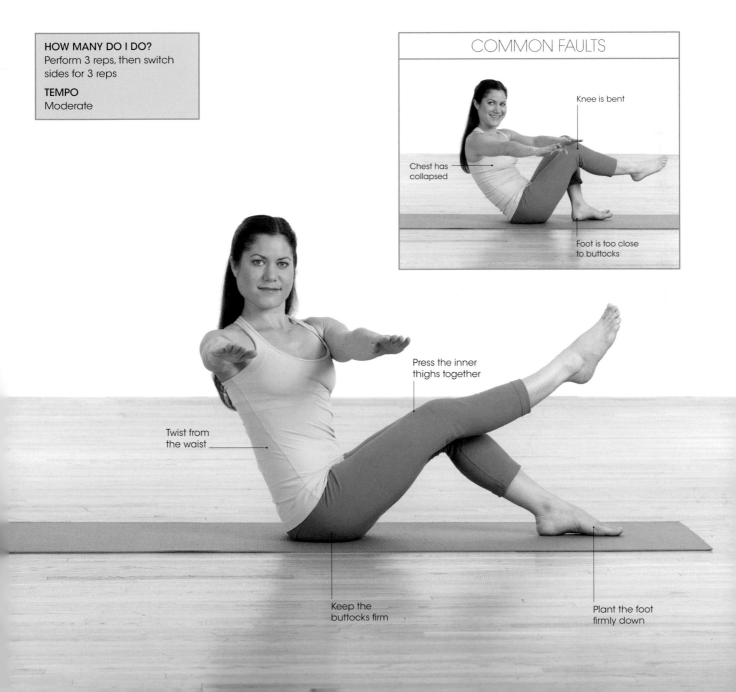

COMMON FAULTS

Knee is bent

Chest has collapsed

Foot is too close to buttocks

Press the inner thighs together

Twist from the waist

Keep the buttocks firm

Plant the foot firmly down

Swimming
Focus on flow

Reciprocal or alternating movements are required for everyday activities like walking. Swimming should be performed with strong attention paid to symmetry and opposition. Focus on working both sides of the body equally.

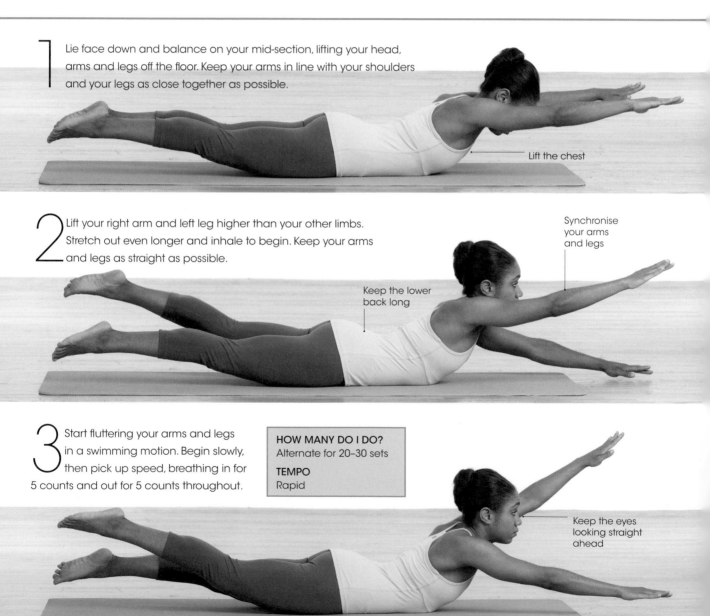

1 Lie face down and balance on your mid-section, lifting your head, arms and legs off the floor. Keep your arms in line with your shoulders and your legs as close together as possible.

Lift the chest

2 Lift your right arm and left leg higher than your other limbs. Stretch out even longer and inhale to begin. Keep your arms and legs as straight as possible.

Synchronise your arms and legs

Keep the lower back long

3 Start fluttering your arms and legs in a swimming motion. Begin slowly, then pick up speed, breathing in for 5 counts and out for 5 counts throughout.

HOW MANY DO I DO?
Alternate for 20–30 sets

TEMPO
Rapid

Keep the eyes looking straight ahead

Down Stretch
Focus on breath

There are a few historical variations of this exercise but the goal is the same for all of them – to open the chest and increase lung capacity at the same time as strengthening the upper back. This version will also tone up your arms.

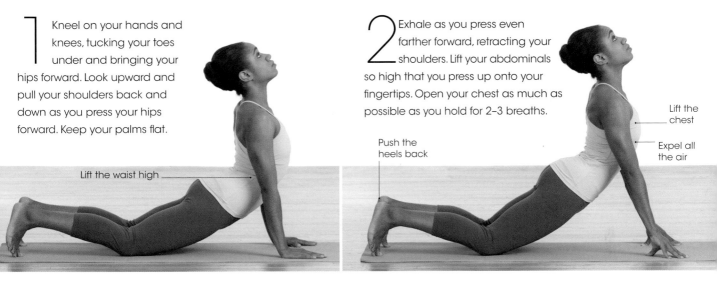

1 Kneel on your hands and knees, tucking your toes under and bringing your hips forward. Look upward and pull your shoulders back and down as you press your hips forward. Keep your palms flat.

Lift the waist high

2 Exhale as you press even farther forward, retracting your shoulders. Lift your abdominals so high that you press up onto your fingertips. Open your chest as much as possible as you hold for 2–3 breaths.

Lift the chest

Push the heels back

Expel all the air

3 Inhale, tuck your head down and press your hips up. Straighten your legs as you rise up on your toes. Allow your palms to lower back down. To repeat, exhale to bend your knees and come down to Step 1.

Keep the lower back long

Tighten the leg muscles

Hang the head between the arms

Press the palms flat

HOW MANY DO I DO?
Perform 4 reps

TEMPO
Slow

Snake
Focus on centring

Snake is an advanced move when performed on the Pilates Reformer machine. Here we combine the benefits of exercises like yoga planks and gymnastic pikes. Your core should drive the movement, so don't rely just on your arms and legs.

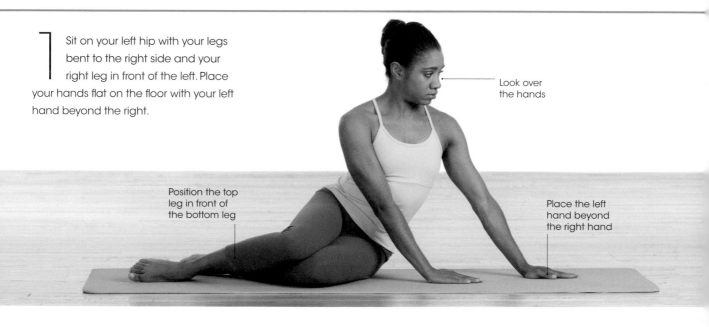

1 Sit on your left hip with your legs bent to the right side and your right leg in front of the left. Place your hands flat on the floor with your left hand beyond the right.

Look over the hands

Position the top leg in front of the bottom leg

Place the left hand beyond the right hand

2 Breathe in with the air and in one single movement, lift your hips and twist until you are facing the floor. Support yourself on your hands and tiptoes. Draw your navel to your spine.

Keep the head down

Raise the heels up high

Swivel the feet so they are parallel

3 Lift your head and lower your hips to bring your body into a snake-like arch. Exhale or "hiss" the air out.

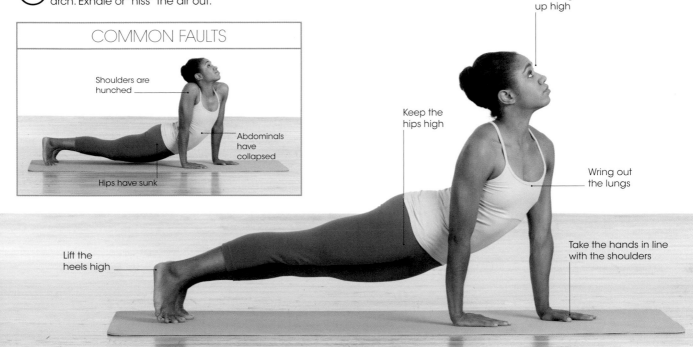

COMMON FAULTS

Shoulders are hunched

Abdominals have collapsed

Hips have sunk

Lift the gaze up high

Keep the hips high

Wring out the lungs

Lift the heels high

Take the hands in line with the shoulders

4 Inhale to return to Step 2, dropping your head down and lifting your hips up. Return to your Step 1 starting position by bending your knees and lowering your left hip to the mat. Repeat before switching to the other side.

HOW MANY DO I DO?
Perform 3–5 reps, then switch sides for 3–5 reps

TEMPO
Moderate

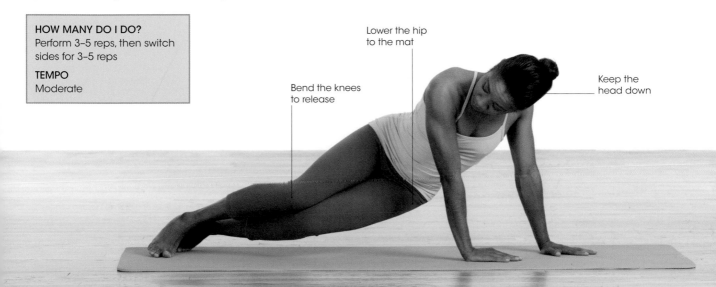

Lower the hip to the mat

Keep the head down

Bend the knees to release

Elephant
Focus on concentration

Elephant is our transition to standing and allows us to finish our programme upright.
I insist that my clients finish their sessions standing upright so they can go straight
from their Pilates work into their everyday activities.

1 Stand with the palms of your hands
flat on the floor so your body forms
an inverted "V". Straighten your knees
as much as possible and pull your abs up
very high (see p.61). Tuck your head down
between your arms and inhale to begin.

Lift the
waist in
and up

Picture yourself
from underneath

2 Exhale as you walk your right foot in one
step towards your hands. Keep your
knees as straight as possible and lift your
right hip to help advance your foot. Then step
your left foot forward in the same way. Take full
deep breaths as you keep walking until your feet
are between your hands. Drop your head and
fold your body in half. Keep the lift in the abs.
Walk back out to your starting position to repeat.

Aim the chest
towards the knees

Extend the head
towards the shin

Flex the feet clear
of the floor

HOW MANY DO I DO?
Perform 2–3 reps

TEMPO
Slow

Leg Swings: Front
Focus on precision

Ending your workouts with a final spike in your heart rate helps speed your metabolism. Rather than work all of the finer points of Pilates in this exercise, think just of moving freely. Your body is training for real life, so moving in a natural way will serve you well.

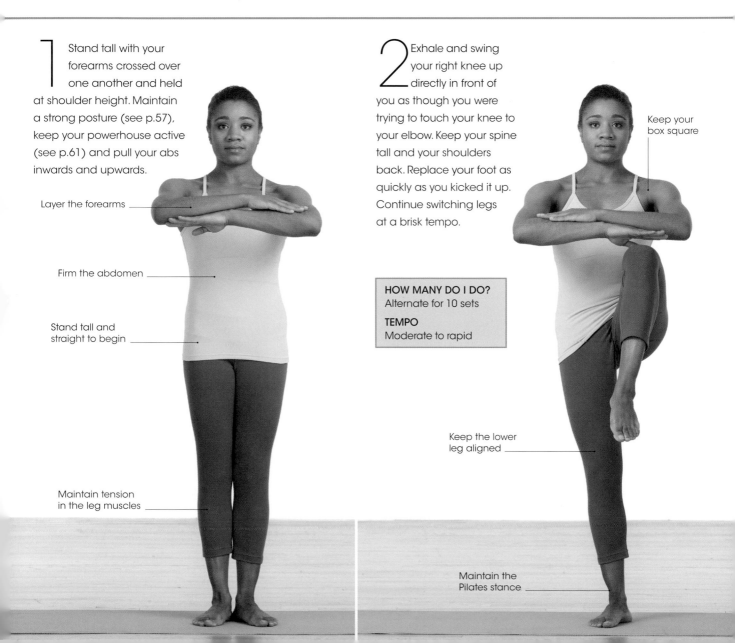

1 Stand tall with your forearms crossed over one another and held at shoulder height. Maintain a strong posture (see p.57), keep your powerhouse active (see p.61) and pull your abs inwards and upwards.

Layer the forearms

Firm the abdomen

Stand tall and straight to begin

Maintain tension in the leg muscles

2 Exhale and swing your right knee up directly in front of you as though you were trying to touch your knee to your elbow. Keep your spine tall and your shoulders back. Replace your foot as quickly as you kicked it up. Continue switching legs at a brisk tempo.

Keep your box square

Keep the lower leg aligned

Maintain the Pilates stance

HOW MANY DO I DO?
Alternate for 10 sets

TEMPO
Moderate to rapid

Leg Swings: Side
Focus on control

Tight hips eventually cause all kinds of problems in the joints, not to mention wear and tear on your spine. Leg Swings: Side will open the hips and work the muscles in that area to prevent poor body mechanics and improve your ease of movement.

1 Stand with your heels together, toes apart and arms held out to the sides.
Take your palms face down.
Pull your abs in and up.

2 Inhale to prepare, then exhale as you kick your right knee up sideways, aiming it at your right elbow. Lower the leg. Continue, switching legs and increasing the height and energy of your leg swings each time. Keep your body strong and still throughout.

> **HOW MANY DO I DO?**
> Alternate for 10 sets
> **TEMPO**
> Moderate to rapid

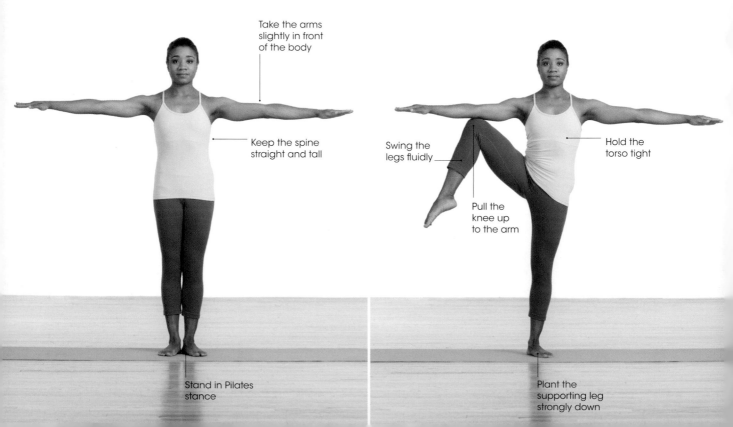

Take the arms slightly in front of the body

Keep the spine straight and tall

Stand in Pilates stance

Swing the legs fluidly

Pull the knee up to the arm

Hold the torso tight

Plant the supporting leg strongly down

Round the World I
Focus on centring

Abdominal muscles have to work in many different directions at the same time all day long. And they have to do all of that while you are upright. Train your muscles to work the way they were meant to with this standing version of Round the World.

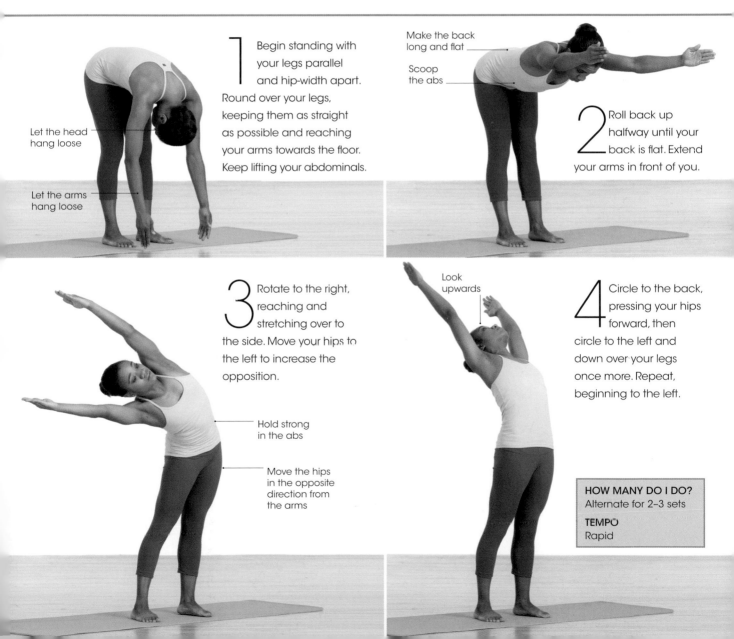

1 Begin standing with your legs parallel and hip-width apart. Round over your legs, keeping them as straight as possible and reaching your arms towards the floor. Keep lifting your abdominals.

Let the head hang loose

Let the arms hang loose

Make the back long and flat

Scoop the abs

2 Roll back up halfway until your back is flat. Extend your arms in front of you.

3 Rotate to the right, reaching and stretching over to the side. Move your hips to the left to increase the opposition.

Hold strong in the abs

Move the hips in the opposite direction from the arms

Look upwards

4 Circle to the back, pressing your hips forward, then circle to the left and down over your legs once more. Repeat, beginning to the left.

HOW MANY DO I DO?
Alternate for 2–3 sets

TEMPO
Rapid

15-minute sequence

Welcome to the first Intermediate programme. Some of these exercises are familiar from the Beginner sequence but incorporate small changes. Just because you have some experience now, don't speed through the workout. Move precisely for best results.

1 Ten by Ten
p.112
Perform 100 pumps
Come up to sitting for no 2

2 Half Roll-Up
p.113
Perform 5 reps
Lie back on your mat
for no 3

3 Mini Bridge
p.114
Perform 3 reps
Sit up towards the front
of your mat for no 4

4 Rolling Like a Ball II
p.115
Perform 8–10 reps
Lie flat on your back
for no 5

5 Single Leg Stretch II
p.118
Alternate for 8–10 sets
Stay flat on your back for no 6

6 Double Leg Stretch II
p.119
Perform 6–8 reps
Sit up tall for no 7

7 Spine Stretch Forward II
p.121
Perform 5 reps
Stay seated upright
for no 8

8 Round Back
p.124
Perform 5 reps
Remain seated for
no 9

9 Side to Side
p.126
Alternate for 3 sets
Roll onto your left
side for no 10

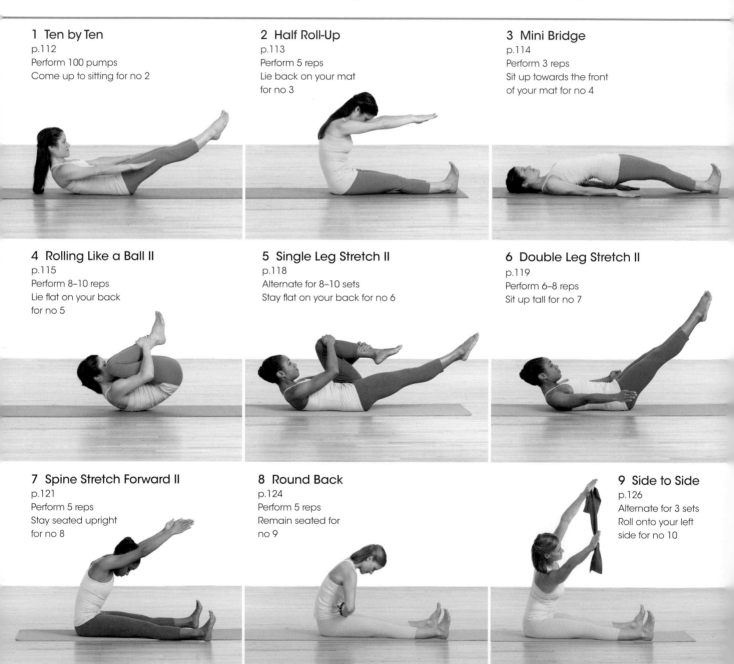

10 Side Kicks: Front II p.130
Perform 10 kicks front and back
Remain on your side for no 11

11 Side Kicks: Circles p.132
Perform 10 circles in each direction,
then change sides and repeat
numbers 10 and 11 on your right side
Come onto all fours for no 12

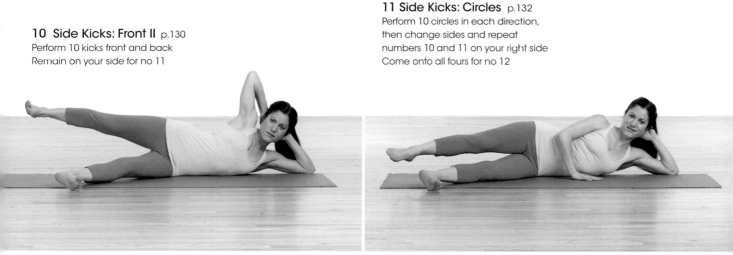

12 Down Stretch
p.139
Perform 4 reps
Stand up with your
hands flat on the floor
for no 13

**14 Round the
World I** p.145
Alternate for 2–3 sets

13 Elephant p.142
Perform 2–3 reps
Stand up tall for
no 14

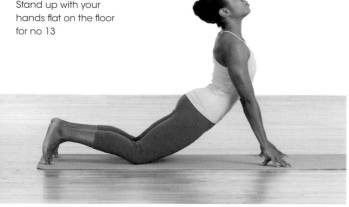

30-minute sequence

This 30-minute Intermediate programme marks your arrival at the halfway point of all the programmes in this book. This is a hallmark workout in your practice. Take your time here before progressing to the next workout.

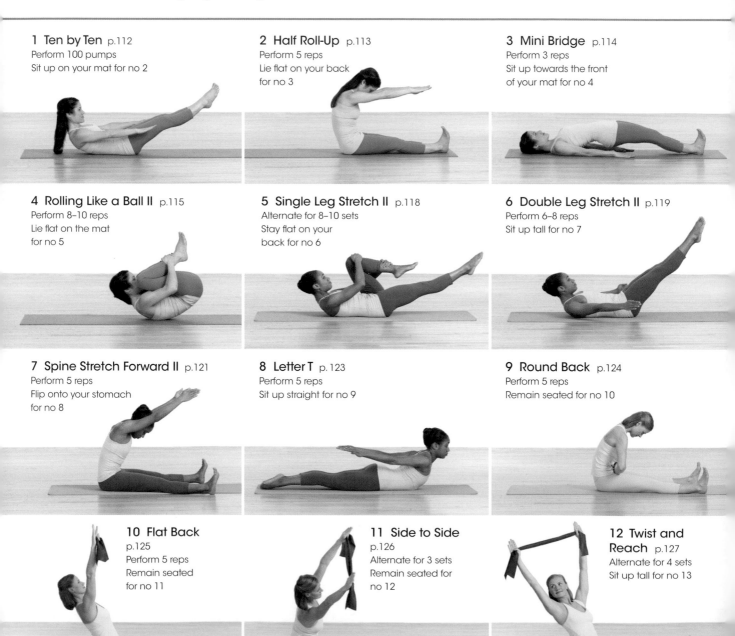

1 Ten by Ten p.112
Perform 100 pumps
Sit up on your mat for no 2

2 Half Roll-Up p.113
Perform 5 reps
Lie flat on your back
for no 3

3 Mini Bridge p.114
Perform 3 reps
Sit up towards the front
of your mat for no 4

4 Rolling Like a Ball II p.115
Perform 8–10 reps
Lie flat on the mat
for no 5

5 Single Leg Stretch II p.118
Alternate for 8–10 sets
Stay flat on your
back for no 6

6 Double Leg Stretch II p.119
Perform 6–8 reps
Sit up tall for no 7

7 Spine Stretch Forward II p.121
Perform 5 reps
Flip onto your stomach
for no 8

8 Letter T p.123
Perform 5 reps
Sit up straight for no 9

9 Round Back p.124
Perform 5 reps
Remain seated for no 10

10 Flat Back p.125
Perform 5 reps
Remain seated
for no 11

11 Side to Side p.126
Alternate for 3 sets
Remain seated for
no 12

12 Twist and Reach p.127
Alternate for 4 sets
Sit up tall for no 13

13 Neck Pull p.128

Perform 5 reps
Lie on your left side for no 14

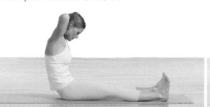

14 Side Kicks: Front II p.130

Perform 10 kicks front and back
Remain on your side for no 15

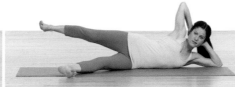

15 Side Kicks: Scissors p.131

Perform 18 kicks back and forth
Remain on your side for no 16

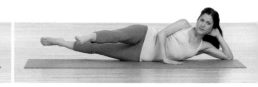

16 Side Kicks: Circles p.132

Perform 10 circles in each direction, then change sides and repeat numbers 14, 15 and 16 on your right side
Sit up tall for no 17

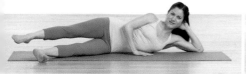

17 Backward Teaser pp.134–5

Perform 4–6 reps
Flip onto your stomach for no 18

18 Swimming p.138

Alternate for 20–30 sets
Come onto all fours for no 19

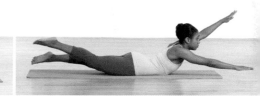

19 Down Stretch p.139

Perform 4 reps
Sit on one hip with legs to one side for no 20

20 Snake pp.140–41

Perform 3–5 reps, then switch sides for 3–5 reps
Stand up with your hands flat on the floor for no 21

21 Elephant p.142

Perform 2–3 reps
Stand up tall for no 22

22 Leg Swings: Front p.143

Alternate for 10 sets
Keep standing tall for no 23

23 Leg Swings: Side p.144

Alternate for 10 sets
Keep standing tall for no 24

24 Round the World I p.145

Alternate for 2–3 sets

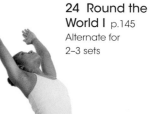

45-minute sequence

Once you reach this routine, you'll have mastered the entire Intermediate programme. This means you're an advanced–intermediate student. When you've memorised this programme, work on flowing smoothly between exercises, making your transitions seamless.

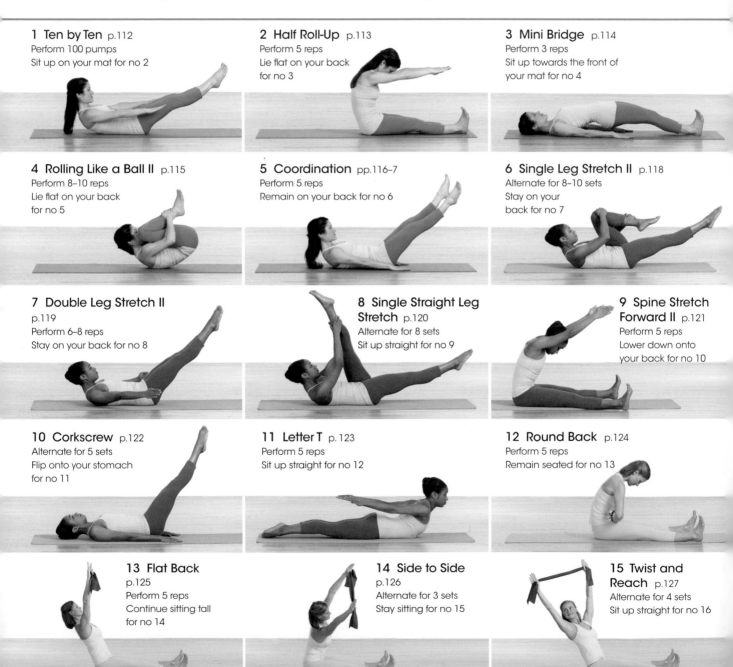

1 Ten by Ten p.112
Perform 100 pumps
Sit up on your mat for no 2

2 Half Roll-Up p.113
Perform 5 reps
Lie flat on your back
for no 3

3 Mini Bridge p.114
Perform 3 reps
Sit up towards the front of
your mat for no 4

4 Rolling Like a Ball II p.115
Perform 8–10 reps
Lie flat on your back
for no 5

5 Coordination pp.116–7
Perform 5 reps
Remain on your back for no 6

6 Single Leg Stretch II p.118
Alternate for 8–10 sets
Stay on your
back for no 7

7 Double Leg Stretch II p.119
Perform 6–8 reps
Stay on your back for no 8

8 Single Straight Leg Stretch p.120
Alternate for 8 sets
Sit up straight for no 9

9 Spine Stretch Forward II p.121
Perform 5 reps
Lower down onto
your back for no 10

10 Corkscrew p.122
Alternate for 5 sets
Flip onto your stomach
for no 11

11 Letter T p.123
Perform 5 reps
Sit up straight for no 12

12 Round Back p.124
Perform 5 reps
Remain seated for no 13

13 Flat Back p.125
Perform 5 reps
Continue sitting tall
for no 14

14 Side to Side p.126
Alternate for 3 sets
Stay sitting for no 15

15 Twist and Reach p.127
Alternate for 4 sets
Sit up straight for no 16

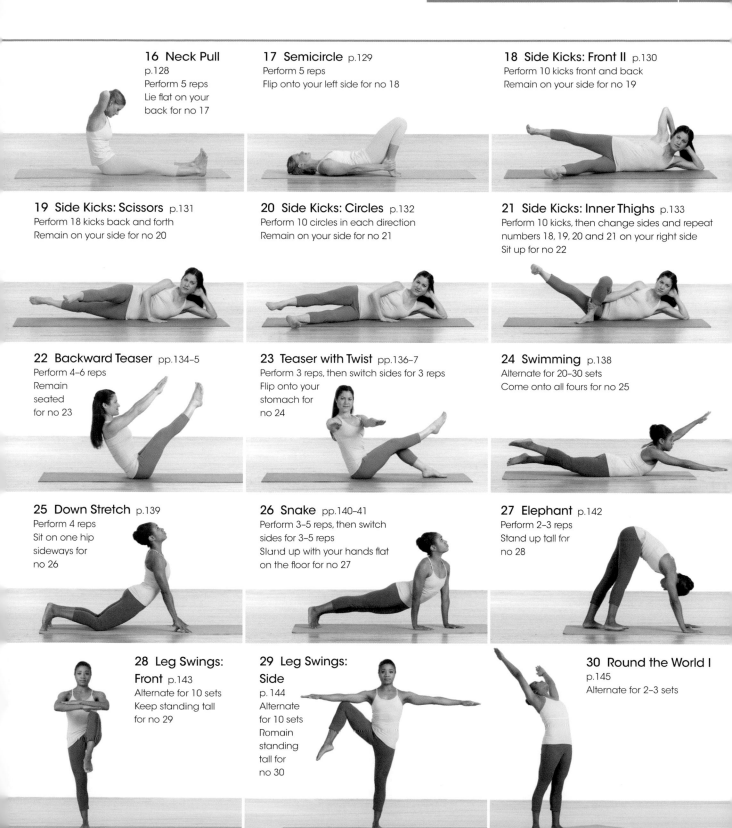

16 Neck Pull p.128
Perform 5 reps
Lie flat on your
back for no 17

17 Semicircle p.129
Perform 5 reps
Flip onto your left side for no 18

18 Side Kicks: Front II p.130
Perform 10 kicks front and back
Remain on your side for no 19

19 Side Kicks: Scissors p.131
Perform 18 kicks back and forth
Remain on your side for no 20

20 Side Kicks: Circles p.132
Perform 10 circles in each direction
Remain on your side for no 21

21 Side Kicks: Inner Thighs p.133
Perform 10 kicks, then change sides and repeat
numbers 18, 19, 20 and 21 on your right side
Sit up for no 22

22 Backward Teaser pp.134–5
Perform 4–6 reps
Remain
seated
for no 23

23 Teaser with Twist pp.136–7
Perform 3 reps, then switch sides for 3 reps
Flip onto your
stomach for
no 24

24 Swimming p.138
Alternate for 20–30 sets
Come onto all fours for no 25

25 Down Stretch p.139
Perform 4 reps
Sit on one hip
sideways for
no 26

26 Snake pp.140–41
Perform 3–5 reps, then switch
sides for 3–5 reps
Stand up with your hands flat
on the floor for no 27

27 Elephant p.142
Perform 2–3 reps
Stand up tall for
no 28

**28 Leg Swings:
Front** p.143
Alternate for 10 sets
Keep standing tall
for no 29

**29 Leg Swings:
Side**
p.144
Alternate
for 10 sets
Remain
standing
tall for
no 30

30 Round the World I
p.145
Alternate for 2–3 sets

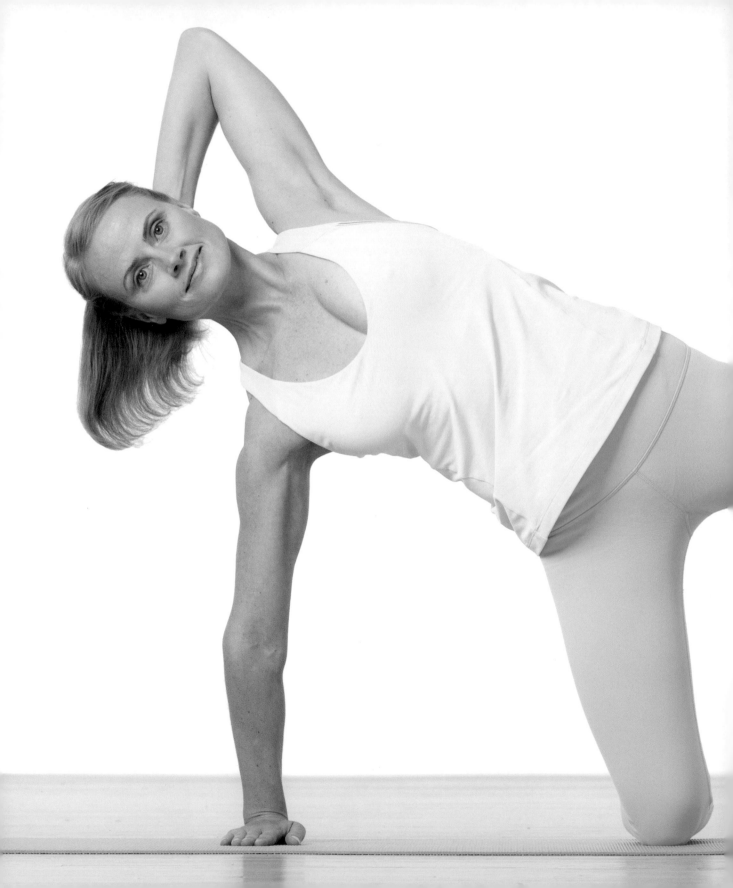

Advanced

There are only two types of students. Beginners
and experienced beginners. You may be taking on
advanced material, but continue to practise
as though you were a new Pilates student.

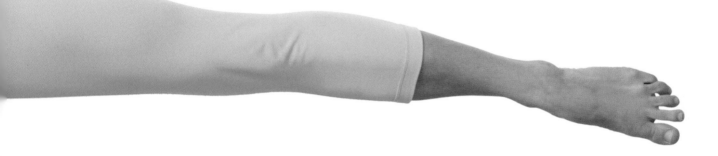

The Hundred
Focus on precision

We begin at the beginning again with the first of the traditional matwork exercises. This time we take our cue from Mr Pilates and his original version of The Hundred. It is a vigorous move that should warm up your entire body quickly.

1 Lie flat on your back with your arms by your sides and your legs pressed together on the mat.

Stretch the arches of the feet long

2 Using your abs, lift your head, legs and feet in one movement. Take your legs and feet 10–15cm (4–6in) off the floor. Stretch your arms forward.

3 Inhale as you pump your arms briskly for 5 pumps, then exhale for another 5 pumps. Continue alternating your breath until you reach 100 pumps. Pause at the end for a final moment, then lower your head, legs and feet with control.

HOW MANY DO I DO?
Perform 10 inhalations and 10 exhalations (100 pumps)

TEMPO
Rapid

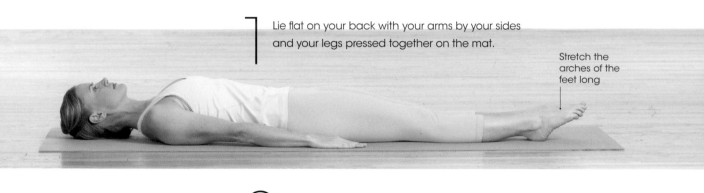

Breathe out through the mouth

Scoop the abs in (see p.61)

Work the glutes

Pump the arms strong and straight

Press the legs together

Hip-Ups
Focus on control

Hip-Ups are an exercise I've devised to prepare the body for overhead movements. It's not the lift that's important here, but the descent. This exercise will reveal how much control you really have and will force you to increase it.

1 Lie flat on your back with your legs up at 90°. Press your arms into the mat by your sides and rotate your legs so your feet form a small "V" with your heels together (Pilates stance, see p.60).

2 Breathing naturally throughout, lift your hips 10–15cm (4–6in), shooting your legs straight up. Hold the lift for a moment, then slowly lower your hips back down to the mat. Repeat 6 times. Rest for a split second before repeating.

HOW MANY DO I DO?
Perform 6 reps, pause briefly, then perform 6 more reps

TEMPO
Moderate to rapid

Stretch the arches of the feet long

Squeeze the backs of the legs

Keep the chest open

Keep the back of the neck long

Work within your frame as you move

Lift the legs straight up

Press the arms into the ground

Lower slowly, rolling through each vertebra (see p.65)

Roll-Over
Focus on precision

This Advanced programme includes some moves that resemble yoga. Roll-Over is a dynamic version of yoga's plough. It's one of the first exercises you'll do that requires you to lift your legs up over your head. Do not rely on momentum. Use your core and control.

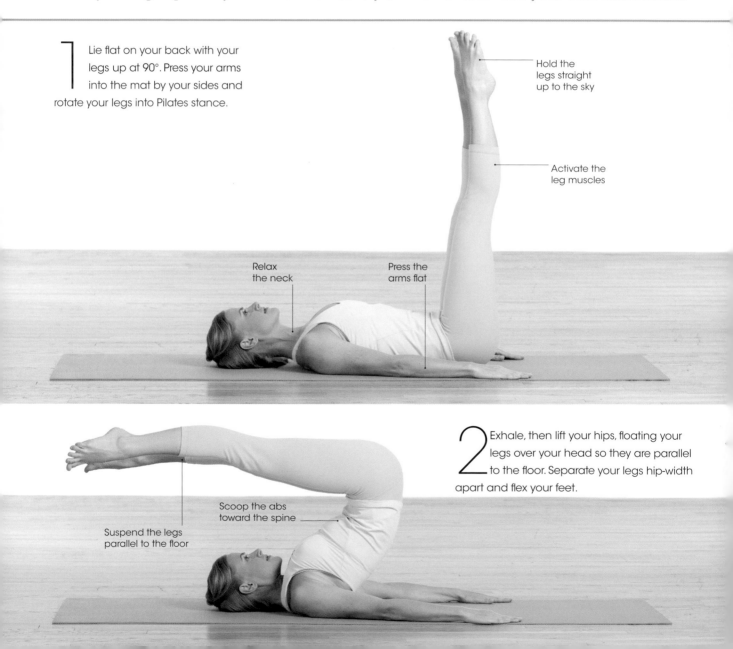

1 Lie flat on your back with your legs up at 90°. Press your arms into the mat by your sides and rotate your legs into Pilates stance.

Hold the legs straight up to the sky

Activate the leg muscles

Relax the neck

Press the arms flat

2 Exhale, then lift your hips, floating your legs over your head so they are parallel to the floor. Separate your legs hip-width apart and flex your feet.

Suspend the legs parallel to the floor

Scoop the abs toward the spine

3 Slowly lower your hips back to the mat with control and resistance (see p.57). Roll through each vertebra, articulating through the entire length of your spine.

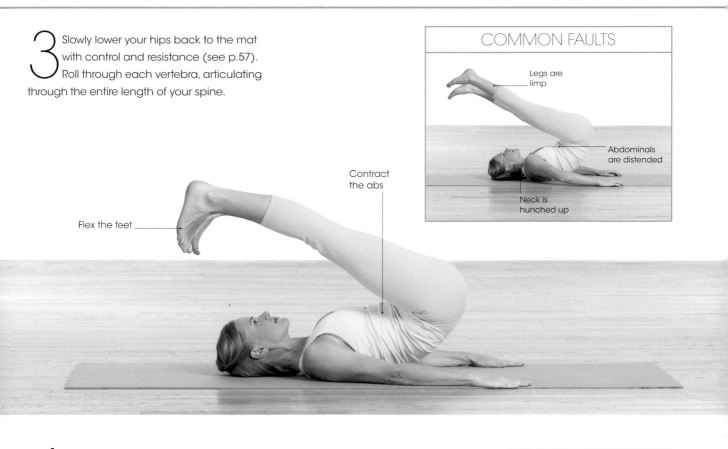

Flex the feet

Contract the abs

COMMON FAULTS

Legs are limp

Abdominals are distended

Neck is hunched up

4 When your spine is flat on the mat again, lower your legs halfway towards the floor, holding tight in your abs. Point your feet, close your legs and swing them up and over to begin again.

HOW MANY DO I DO?
Perform 5 reps

TEMPO
Slow to moderate

Press the heels up

Pull the spine towards the mat

Press the palms flat

Climb a Tree
Focus on centring

Exercise is simply physics. Having one leg up in the air makes a sit-up very difficult. Remember to be your own teacher continually and assess which side of your body may be stronger or weaker, as well as any misalignments you see in yourself.

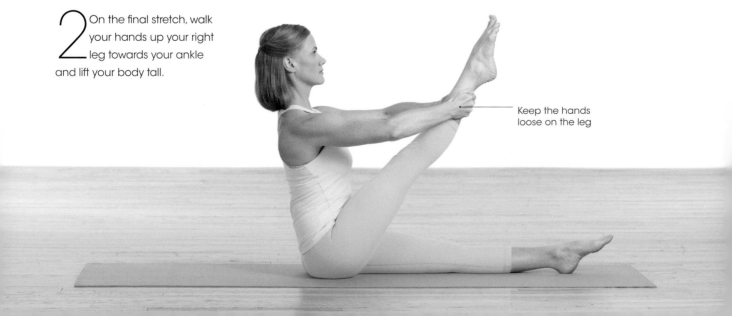

1 Sit upright with your left leg centred on the mat and your right leg bent tightly into your body. Pull your abs in and up, and lift your chest high. Straighten then bend your right leg 3 times.

Hold the leg tight against the body

2 On the final stretch, walk your hands up your right leg towards your ankle and lift your body tall.

Keep the hands loose on the leg

3 Keep your right leg straight up as you lower your back away from it, "walking" yourself down to the mat. Inhale as you lower. Continue until your shoulder blades touch the mat.

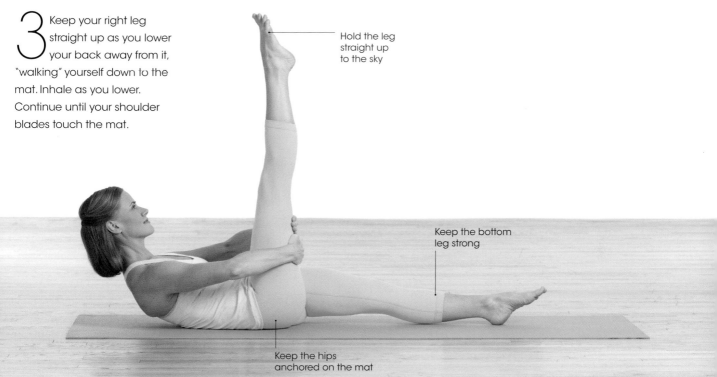

Hold the leg straight up to the sky

Keep the bottom leg strong

Keep the hips anchored on the mat

4 Exhale as you "climb" back up the leg, walking up hand over hand and stretching your body tall when you reach your highest point. Tighten your upper-thigh muscle for an extra stretch. Walk down and climb up twice more before switching legs.

HOW MANY DO I DO?
Perform 3 reps, then switch sides for 3 reps

TEMPO
Moderate

Bring the body to meet the leg

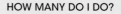

Tighten the thigh to straighten the knee

Rolling Like a Ball III
Focus on flow

Rolling Like a Ball is on the roster once again. You should do a full body roll at least once in your Pilates programme. Practise this variation when you are comfortable with the earlier variations (see p.75 and p.115).

1 Sit with enough room behind you so you can roll back on your mat and with your knees bent tight into your body. Cross your arms round your ankles and grasp the opposite wrist or forearm. Drop your head to begin.

2 Tip back slightly, let your lower back curl towards the floor and pause. As you hold, keep pulling up in your mid-section (see p.57) so you do not collapse. Hold for 3 breaths.

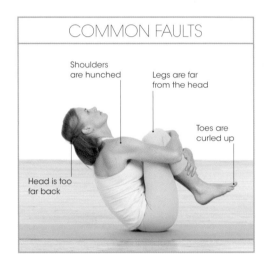

COMMON FAULTS

Shoulders are hunched

Legs are far from the head

Toes are curled up

Head is too far back

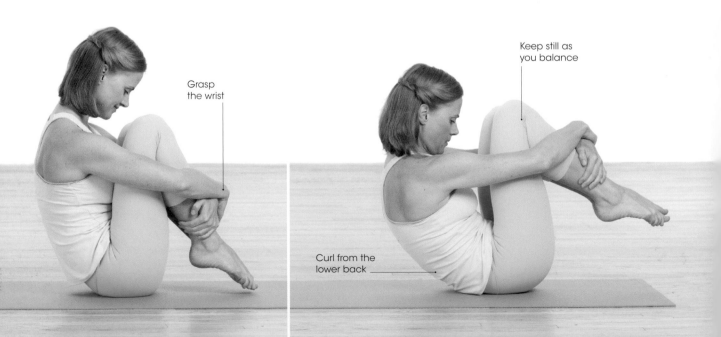

Grasp the wrist

Keep still as you balance

Curl from the lower back

3 Now roll completely upside down, lifting your hips up in the air. Keep your head tucked between your knees the entire time. Your head should not touch the floor when you roll back. Exhale as you roll back up. Use abdominal strength to bring you up with each repetition.

HOW MANY DO I DO?
Perform 8–10 reps

TEMPO
Moderate

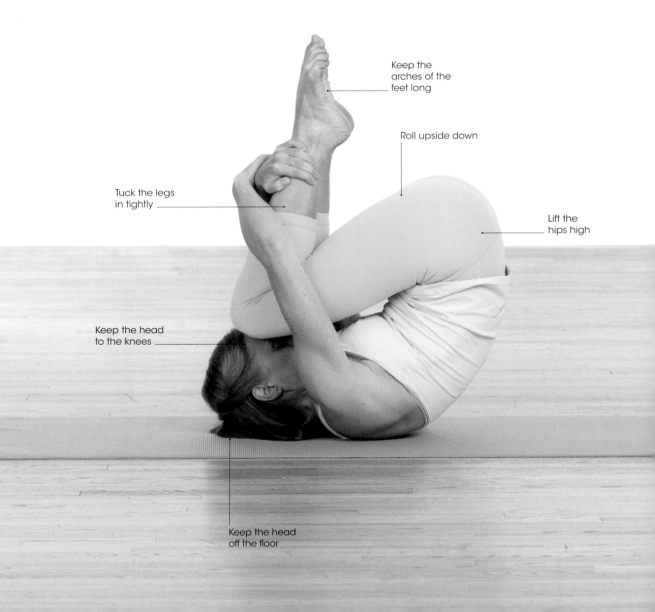

Keep the arches of the feet long

Roll upside down

Tuck the legs in tightly

Lift the hips high

Keep the head to the knees

Keep the head off the floor

Footwork
Focus on control

Teachers often substitute Footwork I for the classic Stomach Series on the mat. Although this may look like a lower-body move, keeping your hands back and your legs pushing outward places a heavy load on the abs – enough to tone and flatten your mid-section.

1 Lie flat on your back with your hands behind your head. Take your knees into your chest, holding them apart but with your feet together like a frog, then curl up into a crunch position (see p.57). Keep your elbows wide and inhale to begin.

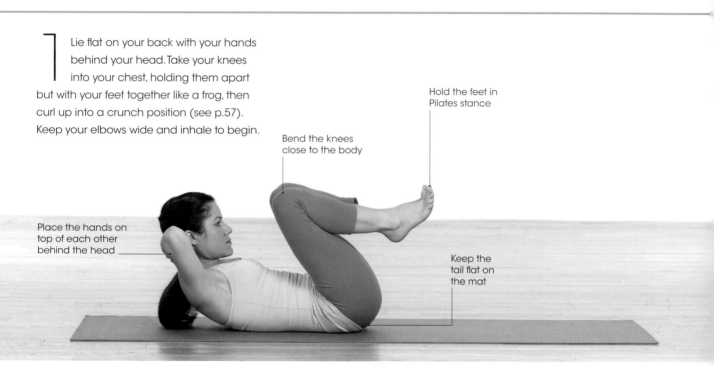

Hold the feet in
Pilates stance

Bend the knees
close to the body

Place the hands on
top of each other
behind the head

Keep the
tail flat on
the mat

2 Hold your body still and exhale to extend your legs straight out on a low diagonal. Continue straightening and bending back in with resistance, keeping your abs scooped in tight. Lower your head to finish.

HOW MANY DO I DO?
Perform 10 reps

TEMPO
Moderate

Use the balls
of the feet to
press out

Anchor the back
to the floor

Keep the shoulders
off the mat

Double Straight Leg Stretch
Focus on centring

Segue into this exercise straight from Footwork I (see opposite). Sequencing in training can often be the key to results. This one-two combo is great for carving out your abs. As you memorise your workout, eliminate any pauses in between moves.

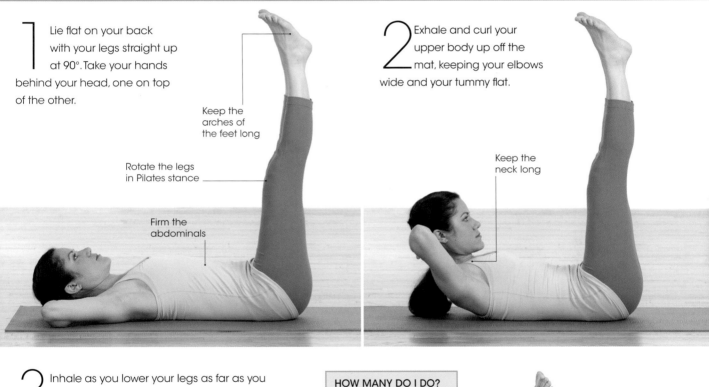

1 Lie flat on your back with your legs straight up at 90°. Take your hands behind your head, one on top of the other.

Keep the arches of the feet long

Rotate the legs in Pilates stance

Firm the abdominals

2 Exhale and curl your upper body up off the mat, keeping your elbows wide and your tummy flat.

Keep the neck long

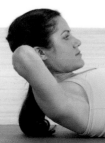

3 Inhale as you lower your legs as far as you can while still holding tight in your abs. Exhale as you pull your legs up for a slow count of 3. Continue with a steady, even tempo.

HOW MANY DO I DO?
Perform 5–8 reps

TEMPO
Slow

Anchor the spine to the mat

Keep the abs scooped

Lift the legs slowly with resistance

Criss-Cross
Focus on precision

Criss-Cross is the icing on the cake of your ab series. This version is one that my Pilates teacher routinely gave me, both when I was a young apprentice and for many years after. Focus on getting and then maintaining your deepest abdominal contraction.

1 Lie flat on your back with both hands behind your head, then bend both knees into your chest. Using your powerhouse (see p.61), curl your upper body up until your shoulders clear the mat.

Layer the hands one on top of the other

2 Exhale and twist left, stretching your right leg out long. Aim your right elbow for your left knee and hold for a count of 3. Look behind you to lift higher and twist more. Anchor your hips to avoid rocking to one side. Inhale to return to the centre and exhale to twist right.

Stay high as you turn

Keep the elbows wide

Take the leg out on a low diagonal

Keep the hips flat

HOW MANY DO I DO?
Alternate for 5–8 sets

TEMPO
Slow

Spine Stretch Forward III
Focus on flow

Spinal articulation and a strong C-curve (see p.63) are so central to Pilates that Spine Stretch Forward is a non-negotiable exercise in most, if not all, Pilates workouts. In this Advanced programme, be sure to curve as far as you can.

1 Sit upright with your legs straight apart, just wider than the mat. Raise your arms in line with your shoulders. Flex your feet and pull your abs in. Inhale to begin.

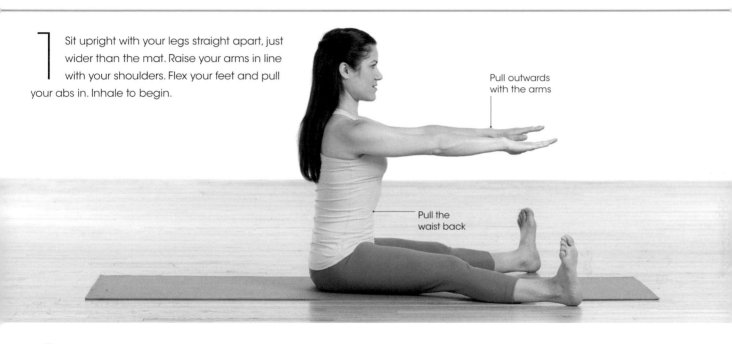

Pull outwards with the arms

Pull the waist back

2 Exhale as you dive forward, rounding your back and pressing your heels away to straighten your legs even more. Use opposition to pull your arms forward and your spine back. Continue exhaling to round even lower, aiming your head to the mat. Inhale to roll up through your spine, one vertebra at a time. Repeat.

HOW MANY DO I DO?
Perform 5 reps

TEMPO
Slow

Duck the head towards the mat

Tighten the leg muscles

Open Leg Rocker
Focus on control

Combine balance, deep core strength, a pinch of timing, a dose of flexibility – and you have Open Leg Rocker. It's easy to rely on momentum in these rolling exercises. Instead, train your muscles to work with strength and control.

1 Sit on your mat with room to roll back and forth. Take hold of your ankles and stretch your legs up straight and just wider than your shoulders. Scoop your abs, lift your chest and inhale deeply.

2 Exhale and, keeping your arms completely straight, curl your tail under, look down and roll backwards until your shoulder blades touch the mat. Keep your head lifted.

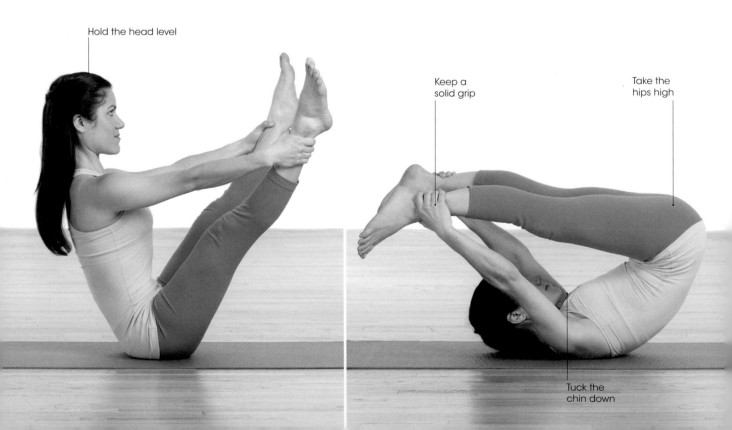

Hold the head level

Keep a solid grip

Take the hips high

Tuck the chin down

3 Inhale at the lowest point of the movement, then exhale and pull your abs in as you roll back up to Step 1. Find your balance then continue rocking. Bend your knees and place your feet flat to finish.

HOW MANY DO I DO?
Perform 8 reps

TEMPO
Moderate

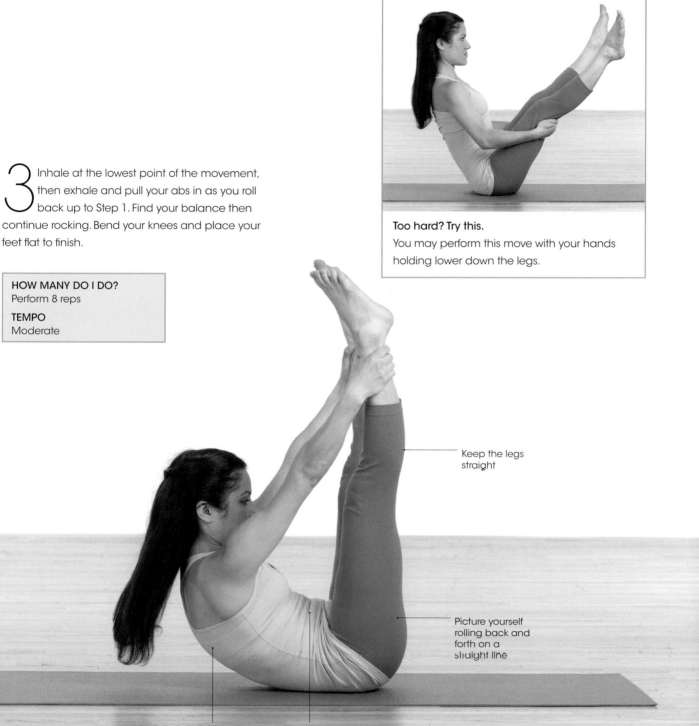

Too hard? Try this.
You may perform this move with your hands holding lower down the legs.

Keep the legs straight

Picture yourself rolling back and forth on a straight line

Roll up smoothly

Contract the abdominals

Corkscrew Overhead
Focus on centring

The beginner Corkscrew (see p.122) trained you to move your legs in a circular pattern with your hips and back flat. To bring you up to the next level and challenge your new-found strength, we will combine the move with a shoulder stand.

1 Lie flat on your back with your legs up at 90°. Press your arms into the mat by your sides and rotate your legs into Pilates stance. Do not use momentum as your legs go overhead.

2 With control, lift your hips and legs up all at once, rising into a shoulder stand. Continue pressing your arms into the floor. Lift your chest but do not crunch your neck.

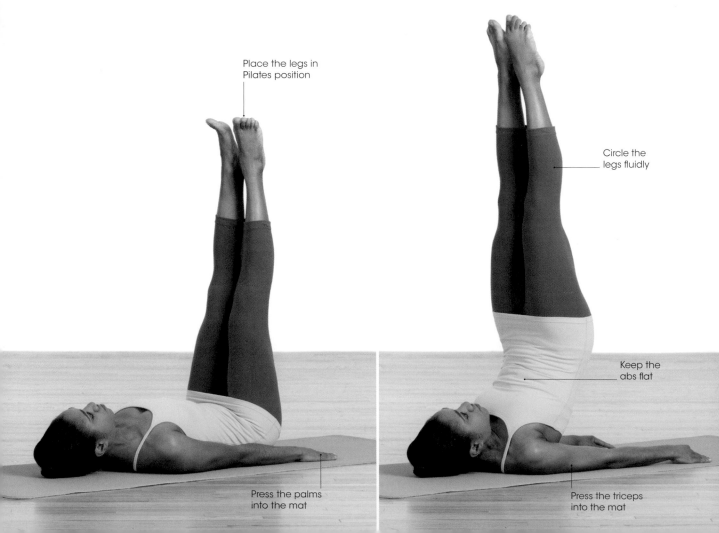

Place the legs in Pilates position

Circle the legs fluidly

Keep the abs flat

Press the palms into the mat

Press the triceps into the mat

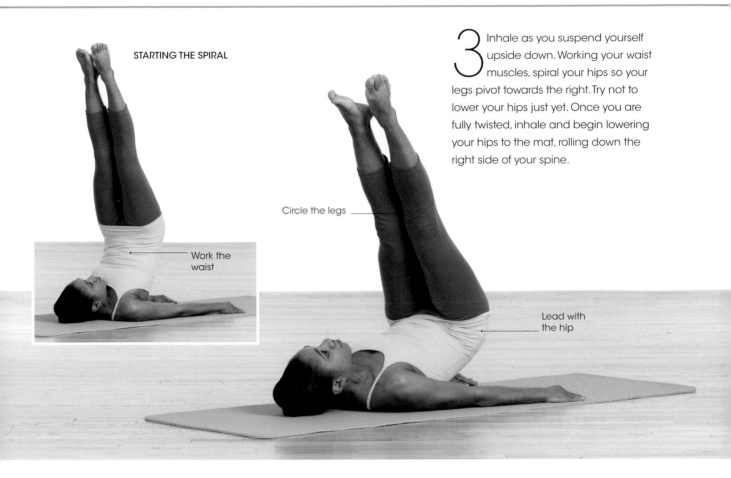

STARTING THE SPIRAL

Work the waist

3 Inhale as you suspend yourself upside down. Working your waist muscles, spiral your hips so your legs pivot towards the right. Try not to lower your hips just yet. Once you are fully twisted, inhale and begin lowering your hips to the mat, rolling down the right side of your spine.

Circle the legs

Lead with the hip

4 Make a controlled descent, lowering one vertebra at a time. As your hips touch down on the right side, exhale and sweep your legs down and over to the left side. Rise right back up on your shoulders as in Step 2 to complete the corkscrew. Switch sides to repeat.

HOW MANY DO I DO?
Alternate for 3 sets

TEMPO
Moderate

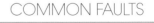

Lower the legs to the right

Keep the feet in Pilates stance

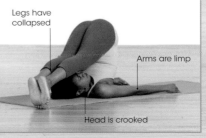

COMMON FAULTS

Legs have collapsed

Arms are limp

Head is crooked

Saw

Focus on breath

Twisting and stretching simultaneously really makes you "wring" your lungs out and gives you an opportunity to work on your breathing technique. Listen carefully to your breathing as you perform this move.

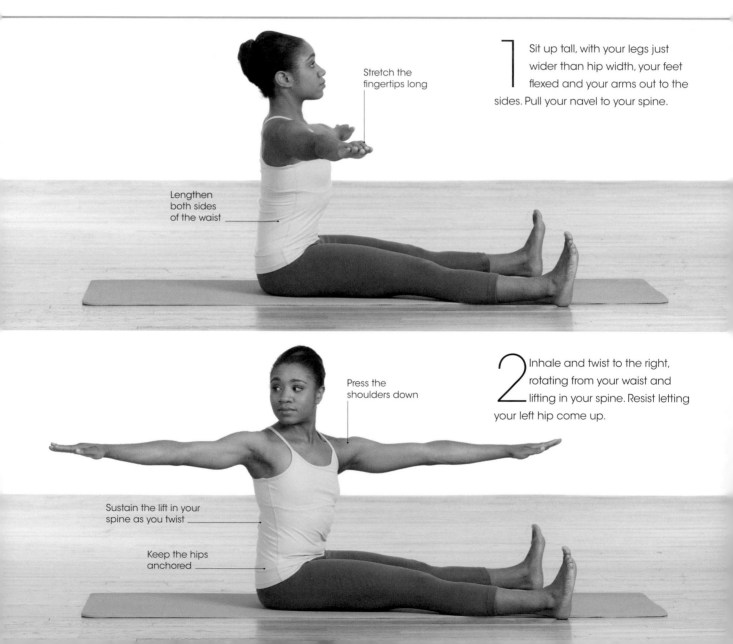

Stretch the fingertips long

1 Sit up tall, with your legs just wider than hip width, your feet flexed and your arms out to the sides. Pull your navel to your spine.

Lengthen both sides of the waist

Press the shoulders down

2 Inhale and twist to the right, rotating from your waist and lifting in your spine. Resist letting your left hip come up.

Sustain the lift in your spine as you twist

Keep the hips anchored

3 Exhale and dive forward, "sawing" off your right little toe as you reach your left hand to the outside of your right foot. Let your head hang and reach your right arm up. Exhale as you twist more, reaching your left ribs towards your right leg. Roll back up to centre and switch sides.

HOW MANY DO I DO?
Alternate for 4 sets

TEMPO
Slow

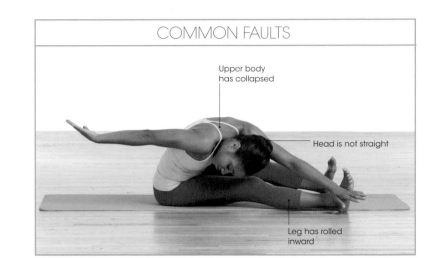

COMMON FAULTS

Upper body has collapsed

Head is not straight

Leg has rolled inward

Stretch the back arm up

Turn the arm so the thumb faces the floor

Keep the opposite hip flat

Expel the air to reach forward

Point the toes straight up

Point the knees straight up

Swan
Focus on flow

A true Pilates original, Swan is lifted straight off the pages of Mr Pilates' book. Overcoming inertia involves an act of strength. Swan will build that strength. For best results, be sure to begin from a static or still position.

1 Lie face down on the mat and lift your upper body just above the mat. Keep your legs and feet on the mat, pressed together tightly. Keep your lower back lengthened. Stretch your arms out to the sides in front of your shoulders and flip your palms upwards.

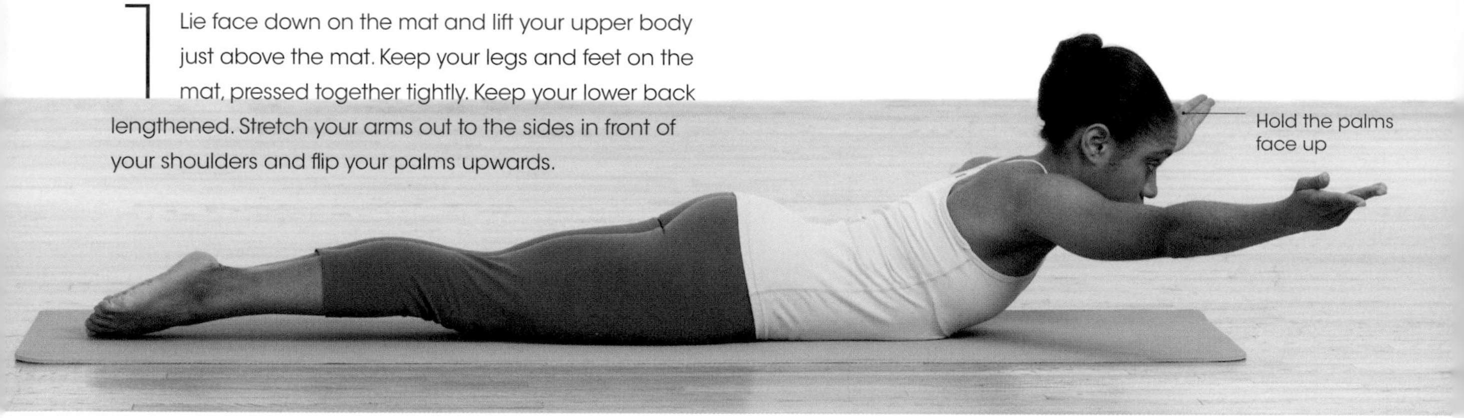

Hold the palms face up

2 Breathing naturally, begin a small forward and back rocking motion. Move smoothly and rhythmically, and make the rocking motion progressively bigger with each repetition.

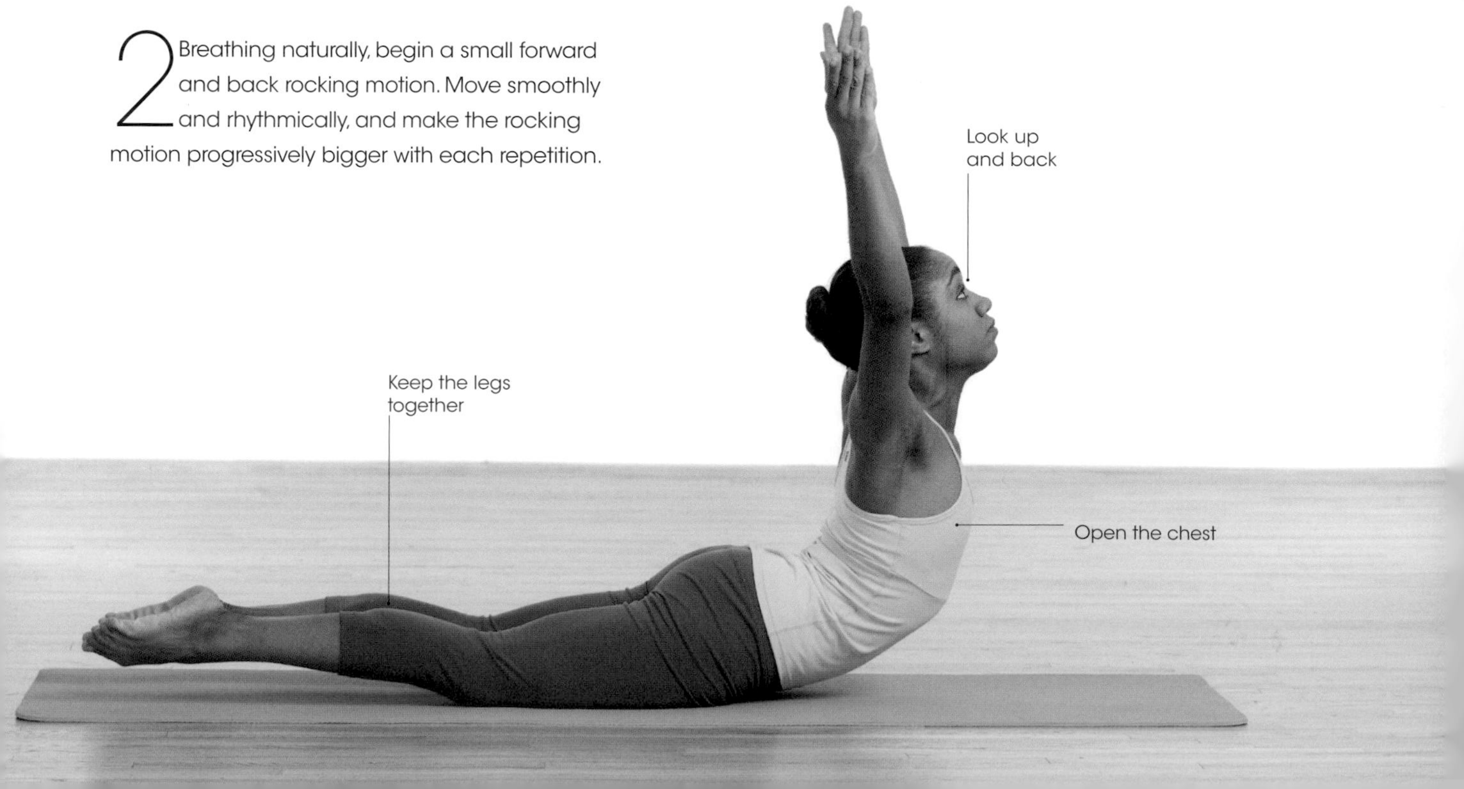

Look up and back

Keep the legs together

Open the chest

3 As you gather momentum, swing your legs up high, which drives your upper body low. Then, all at once, swing your upper body high, driving your legs low.

HOW MANY DO I DO?
Perform 6–10 reps

TEMPO
Moderate

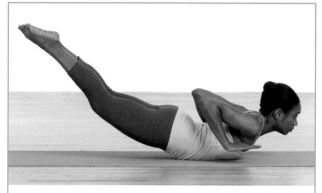

Too hard? Try this.
Use your hands underneath your shoulders to press up. Then release them to swing down repeatedly.

Keep the legs as close together as possible

Turn the palms towards each other

Support the stomach muscles (see p.57)

Keep the chin off the mat

Double Leg Kick
Focus on precision

Double Leg Kick is an exercise in precision. This move will challenge your ability to recruit the targeted muscles by tempting you to recruit muscles that you shouldn't use. Make sure that you are focusing on the correct muscles all the time.

1 Lie face down on your stomach and turn your head to the right. Clasp your hands behind your back and take them as high as they can go between your shoulder blades. Keep your legs together.

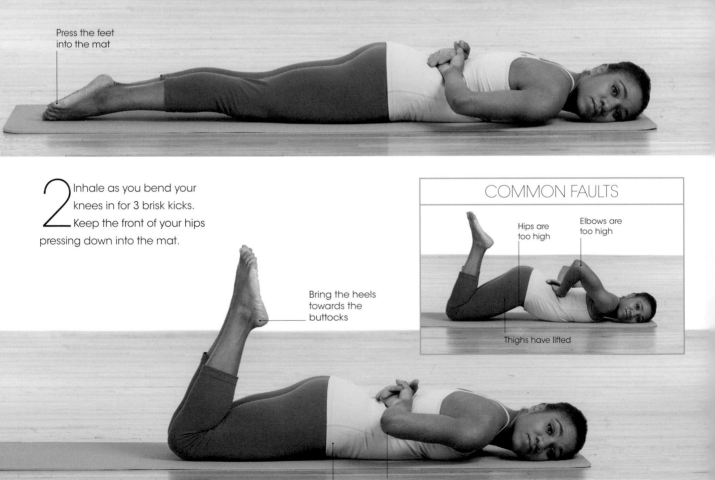

Press the feet into the mat

2 Inhale as you bend your knees in for 3 brisk kicks. Keep the front of your hips pressing down into the mat.

Bring the heels towards the buttocks

COMMON FAULTS

Hips are too high

Elbows are too high

Thighs have lifted

Keep the hips flat

Press the elbows down towards the mat

3 After the third kick, exhale and stretch your legs out long in the air. At the same time, stretch your arms back and pull your body up in a high arc. Keep your abdominals supported and your neck long. Hold for a moment, then lower with control. Return to Step 1, taking your other cheek to the mat to switch sides.

HOW MANY DO I DO?
Alternate for 3 sets

TEMPO
Moderate

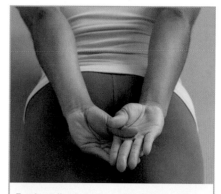

To clasp the hands easily, slide one hand into the palm of the other. When the arms straighten, hook the thumbs together. Keep your fingers stretched.

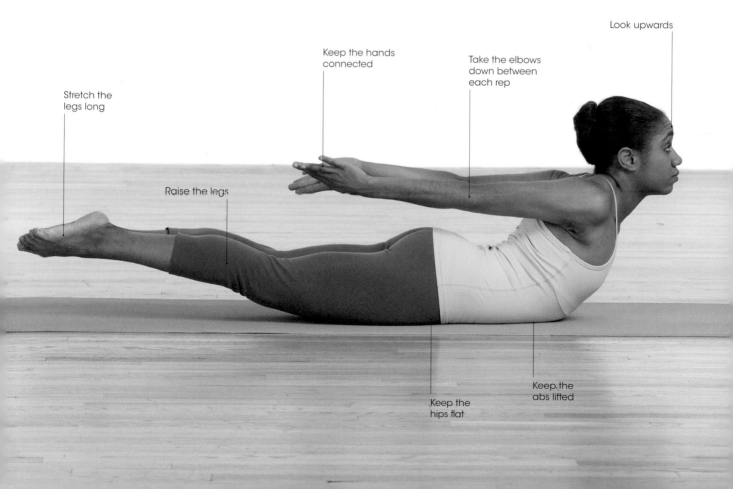

Look upwards

Keep the hands connected

Take the elbows down between each rep

Stretch the legs long

Raise the legs

Keep the hips flat

Keep the abs lifted

Round the World II
Focus on centring

This seated version of Round the World mimics the choreography from the Pilates Reformer more closely than the standing version (see p.145). Exaggerate the motions and angles in this exercise to optimise your results.

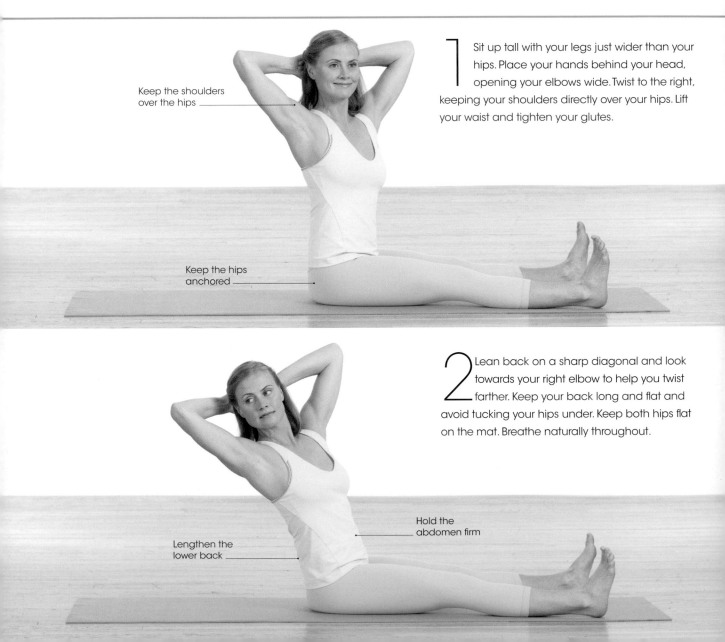

Keep the shoulders over the hips

Keep the hips anchored

1 Sit up tall with your legs just wider than your hips. Place your hands behind your head, opening your elbows wide. Twist to the right, keeping your shoulders directly over your hips. Lift your waist and tighten your glutes.

2 Lean back on a sharp diagonal and look towards your right elbow to help you twist farther. Keep your back long and flat and avoid tucking your hips under. Keep both hips flat on the mat. Breathe naturally throughout.

Hold the abdomen firm

Lengthen the lower back

3 From your farthest point back, keep your right elbow where it is and open the left side of your body until you are straight back, looking upwards. Keep your chest lifted and your tummy flat. Now fold over to the left to complete the Round the World II circuit before returning to upright. Start again, twisting to the left. Continue alternating.

HOW MANY DO I DO?
Alternate for 3 sets

TEMPO
Slow to moderate

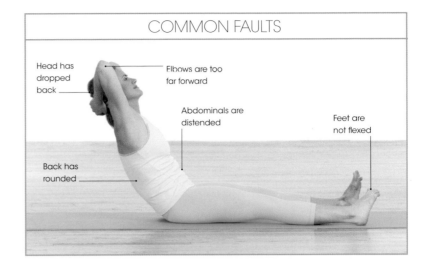

COMMON FAULTS

Head has dropped back

Elbows are too far forward

Abdominals are distended

Feet are not flexed

Back has rounded

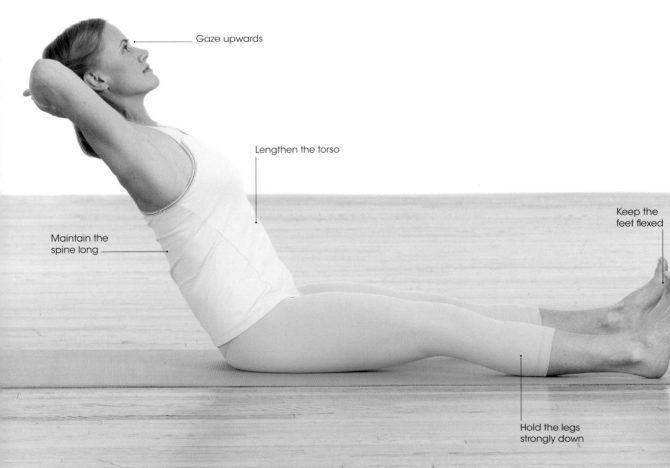

Gaze upwards

Lengthen the torso

Keep the feet flexed

Maintain the spine long

Hold the legs strongly down

Scissors
Focus on concentration

This exercise is taught by many teachers in many different ways. In my opinion, it's always best to start with the original. Study the shapes before beginning the move so you have an image in your mind of what you should look like.

1 Lie flat on your back with your legs up at 90°. Press your arms into the mat by your sides and rotate your legs so your feet form a small "V" with your heels together.

2 Lift your hips as high as possible, raising your legs up straight into a shoulder stand. Place your hands against your lower back for support.

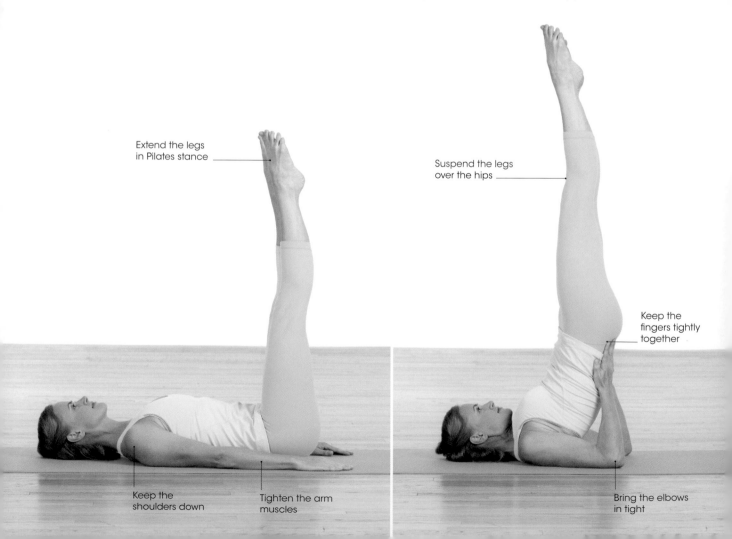

Extend the legs in Pilates stance

Suspend the legs over the hips

Keep the fingers tightly together

Keep the shoulders down

Tighten the arm muscles

Bring the elbows in tight

3 Bring your pelvis down into your hands so your hips lower away from your head. Pause here for a moment to get your balance and fire up your abs (see p.57). Lengthen your waist, compress your abdominals and try to settle your hips into your hands.

4 Breathing naturally, "split" your legs in a scissor-like movement, making a double pulse at the end of the split. Switch legs and keep alternating.

HOW MANY DO I DO?
Alternate for 5 sets
TEMPO
Slow to moderate

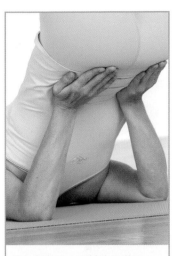

Hand placement is key. Keep the palms flat and the elbows tucked right underneath you.

Keep the arches of the feet long

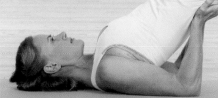

Lower the hips away from the body

Keep space under the chin

Keep the top leg high

Keep the knees straight

Keep the hands flat under the back

Spine Twist II
Focus on flow

Pushing through barriers is something you have to do to improve your physical conditioning. This second version of Spine Twist will make you aware of some of your limits. Persist and fight through it to make gains.

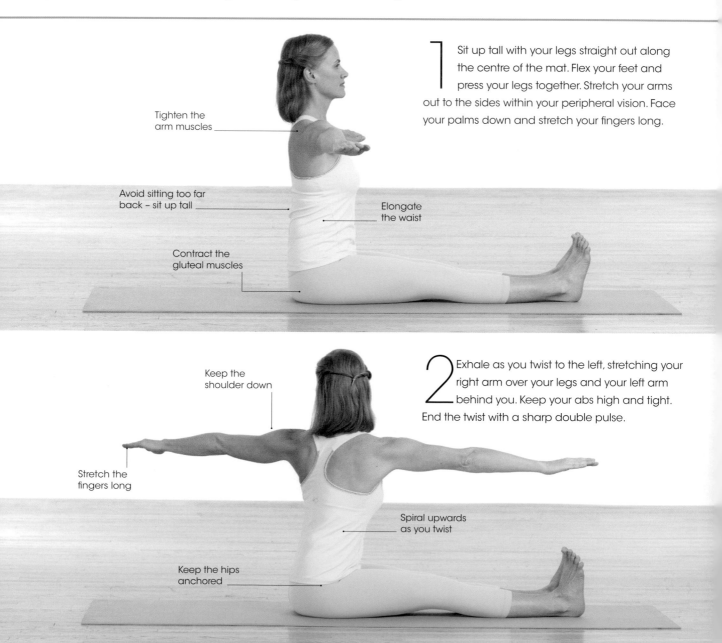

1 Sit up tall with your legs straight out along the centre of the mat. Flex your feet and press your legs together. Stretch your arms out to the sides within your peripheral vision. Face your palms down and stretch your fingers long.

Tighten the arm muscles

Avoid sitting too far back – sit up tall

Contract the gluteal muscles

Elongate the waist

2 Exhale as you twist to the left, stretching your right arm over your legs and your left arm behind you. Keep your abs high and tight. End the twist with a sharp double pulse.

Keep the shoulder down

Stretch the fingers long

Spiral upwards as you twist

Keep the hips anchored

3 Inhale to return to the centre. Exhale to twist to the right. Work your abs with each twist, turning farther and growing taller. Counter any tendency to lean back by pulling forward. Continue alternating.

HOW MANY DO I DO?
Alternate for 5 sets

TEMPO
Moderate to rapid

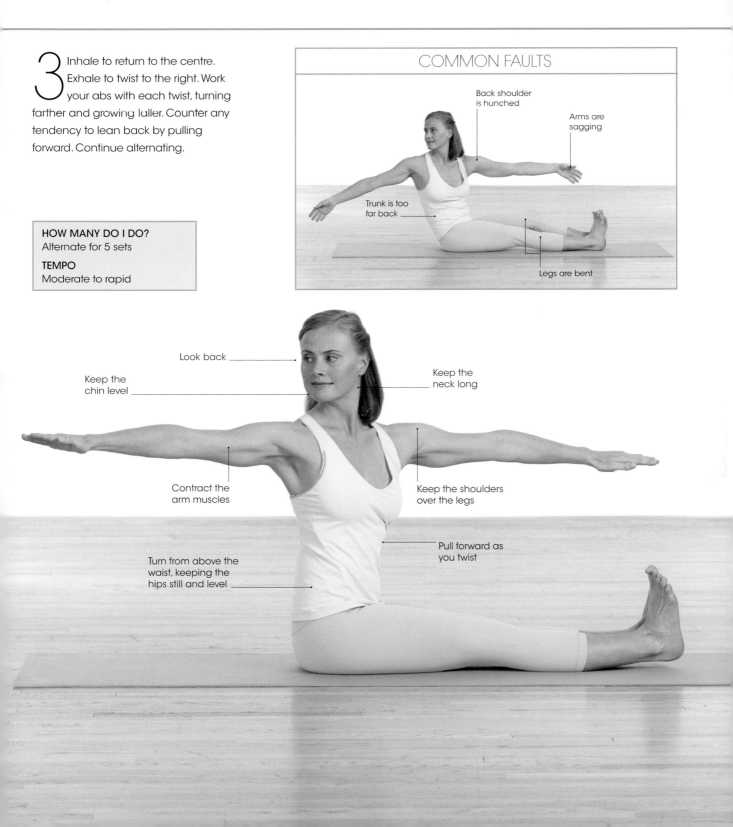

COMMON FAULTS

Back shoulder is hunched

Arms are sagging

Trunk is too far back

Legs are bent

Look back

Keep the chin level

Keep the neck long

Contract the arm muscles

Keep the shoulders over the legs

Pull forward as you twist

Turn from above the waist, keeping the hips still and level

Tendon Stretch
Focus on control

Upper-body work done the way gymnasts do it is a powerful form of training. Tendon Stretch is yet another machine exercise translated to the mat. The result is a high-level movement. Start small and gradually increase your range of motion.

1 Sit upright with both legs extended and pressed together. Flex the feet and place the hands flat on the floor or make them into fists.

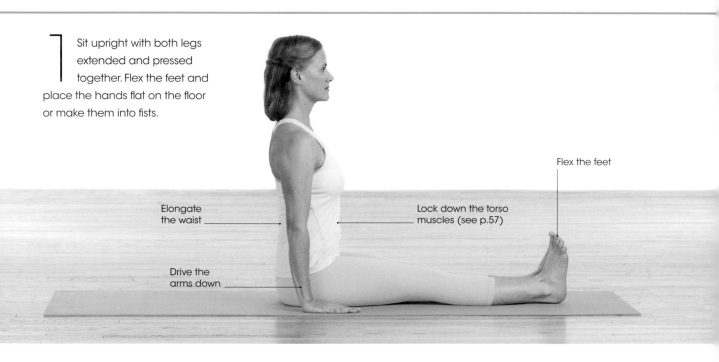

Elongate the waist

Lock down the torso muscles (see p.57)

Flex the feet

Drive the arms down

2 Drop your head, round over your legs and use your upper-body strength and your abs to lift your entire body up off the floor. Pull your hips far back to lift them high.

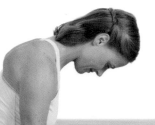

Envisage yourself being pulled backwards

The calves brush the floor

3 Start swinging yourself forward, then back, focusing on the back portion of the swing. To finish, lower your hips to the floor with control, release your hands and rest.

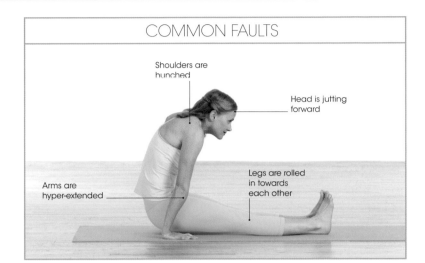

COMMON FAULTS

Shoulders are hunched

Head is jutting forward

Arms are hyper-extended

Legs are rolled in towards each other

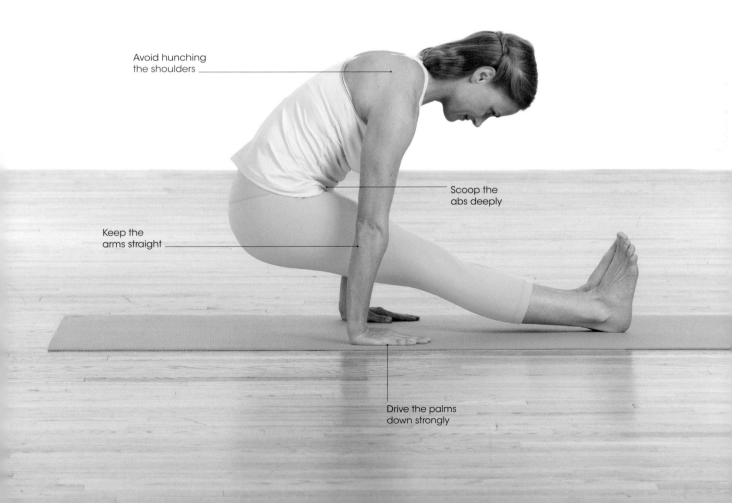

Avoid hunching the shoulders

Scoop the abs deeply

Keep the arms straight

Drive the palms down strongly

Jackknife
Focus on centring

A controlled descent is one of the themes in many of the moves we use in advanced matwork. This is an opportunity to practise that theme and combine it with a big overhead movement. This is a rhythmical exercise with a snappy tempo.

1 Lie flat on your back with your legs up at 90°. Press your arms into the mat by your sides and rotate your legs into Pilates stance.

2 Exhale as you lift your hips up, rolling up high on your shoulders into a shoulder stand. Tighten your buttock muscles and relax your neck and shoulders. Pause a moment.

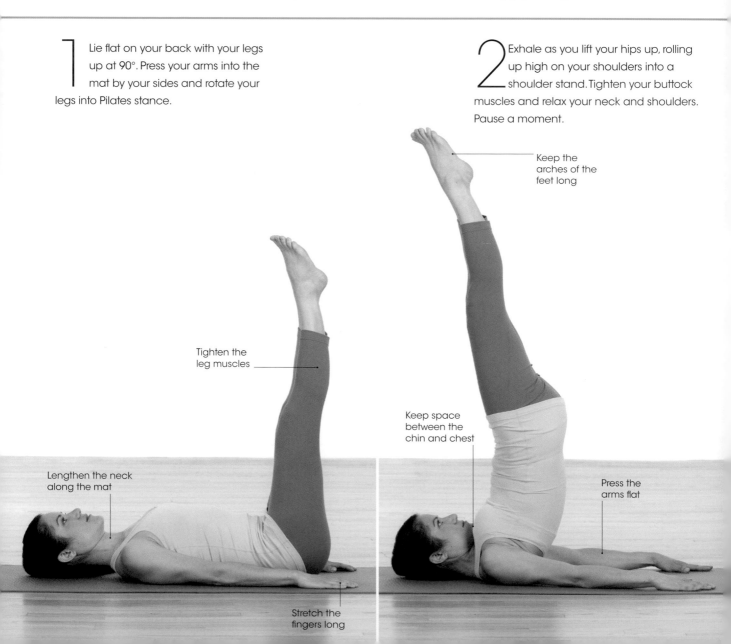

Keep the arches of the feet long

Tighten the leg muscles

Keep space between the chin and chest

Lengthen the neck along the mat

Press the arms flat

Stretch the fingers long

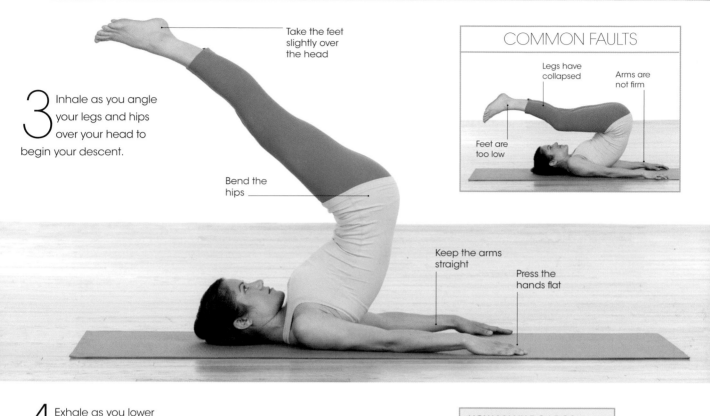

3 Inhale as you angle your legs and hips over your head to begin your descent.

Take the feet slightly over the head

Bend the hips

Keep the arms straight

Press the hands flat

COMMON FAULTS

Legs have collapsed

Arms are not firm

Feet are too low

4 Exhale as you lower your spine vertebra by vertebra, creating resistance as you go. Roll through your middle back, ribs, lower back, then buttocks. End with your legs just below 90°, then repeat.

Keep the feet over the eyes as you lower

Work with resistance

Roll down fluidly, articulating through the spine (see p.57)

HOW MANY DO I DO?
Perform 5 reps

TEMPO
Moderate

Side Kicks: Bicycle
Focus on concentration

One of my Pilates mantras is that no part of an exercise is more important than any other. All are vital to your practice. This side-lying Bicycle has many components, all of which are equally important. Perform all Side Kicks on one side before switching sides.

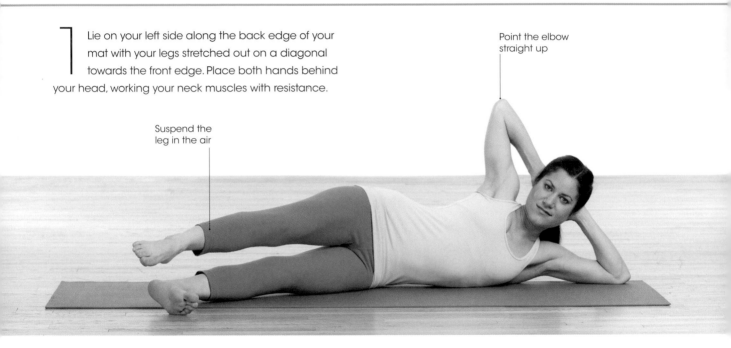

1 Lie on your left side along the back edge of your mat with your legs stretched out on a diagonal towards the front edge. Place both hands behind your head, working your neck muscles with resistance.

Point the elbow straight up

Suspend the leg in the air

2 Holding firm in your powerhouse and inhaling, lift your right leg to hip height and swing it high to the front.

Keep the leg parallel to the floor

Support the abs

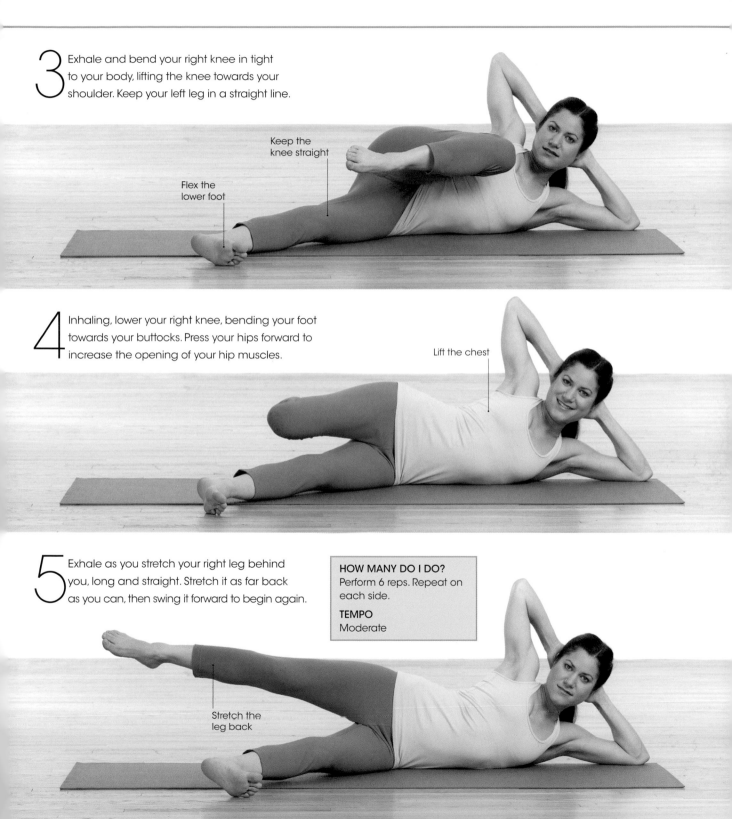

3 Exhale and bend your right knee in tight to your body, lifting the knee towards your shoulder. Keep your left leg in a straight line.

Keep the knee straight

Flex the lower foot

4 Inhaling, lower your right knee, bending your foot towards your buttocks. Press your hips forward to increase the opening of your hip muscles.

Lift the chest

5 Exhale as you stretch your right leg behind you, long and straight. Stretch it as far back as you can, then swing it forward to begin again.

HOW MANY DO I DO?
Perform 6 reps. Repeat on each side.

TEMPO
Moderate

Stretch the leg back

Side Kicks: Rond de Jambe
Focus on precision

The hip joints have a tremendous range of motion, yet we only use them in a limited capacity each day. Rond de Jambe will open and simultaneously strengthen these joints. When you have finished this exercise, repeat from p.186 on your right side.

1 Lie on your left side along the back edge of your mat with your legs stretched out on a diagonal towards the front edge. Support your head on your left hand and either place your right hand behind your head with your left hand or take it to the mat in front of you.

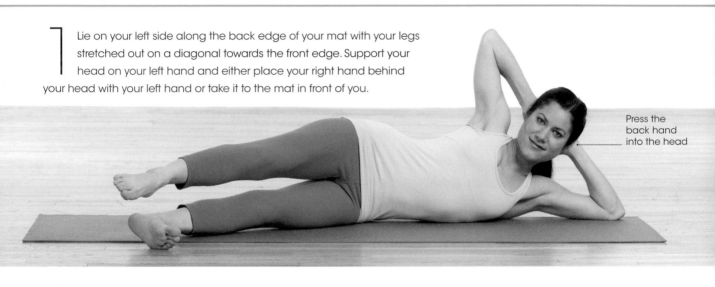

Press the back hand into the head

2 Holding firm in your powerhouse and inhaling, lift your right leg to hip height and carry it forward. Resist the tendency to rock your upper body back.

Keep the shoulders stacked over the hips

Keep the chest high

Take the leg to hip height

3 Exhale and press your hips forward as you rotate your right leg sideways, lifting it up to the ceiling. The sole of your foot should face the sky. Inhale as you stretch your leg higher.

Aim the leg for the ear

Look straight ahead

4 Exhale and lift your right leg back without rocking your body forward. Stretch it as far as it will go. Return your leg to the centre to repeat 2 more times. Reverse direction for 3 reps, starting by swinging your leg back, then taking it up, then forward.

HOW MANY DO I DO?
Perform 3 reps, then reverse direction for 3 reps. Repeat on each side.

TEMPO
Slow to moderate

Keep the hips stacked

Stretch the leg backwards

Teaser III
Focus on flow

This final Teaser is a culmination of your earlier work. In Backward Teaser (see pp.134–5) you practised a controlled descent of your upper body, and in Teaser with Twist (see pp.136–7), of your lower body. Here we put it all together.

1 Lie flat on your back with your arms overhead in line with your ears. Centre your legs on the mat and turn them out slightly so your heels come together. Inhale to begin.

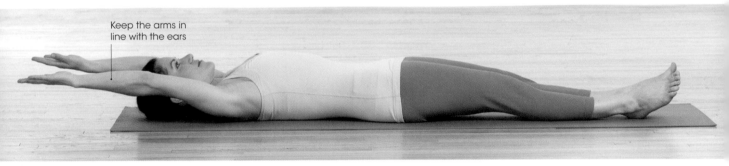

Keep the arms in line with the ears

2 Exhale as you swing your arms and legs up to create a letter "V" with your back and your legs. Stretch your fingers directly over your legs towards your toes. Sit tall, lifting your gaze, chest and waist up very high.

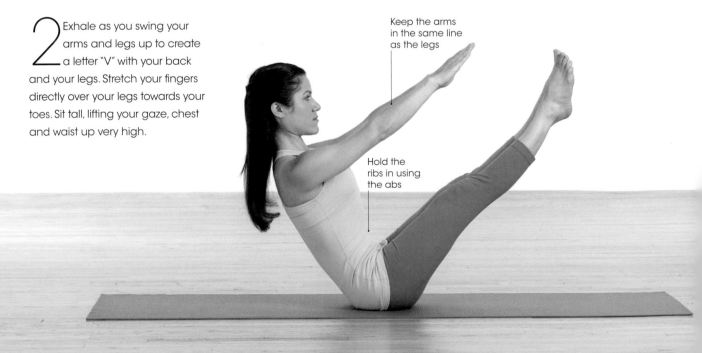

Keep the arms in the same line as the legs

Hold the ribs in using the abs

3 Without disturbing the "V" shape of your lower body, inhale and raise your arms overhead in line with your ears. Pause a moment, then, with resistance, begin to lower your legs and body, keeping your arms stretching back.

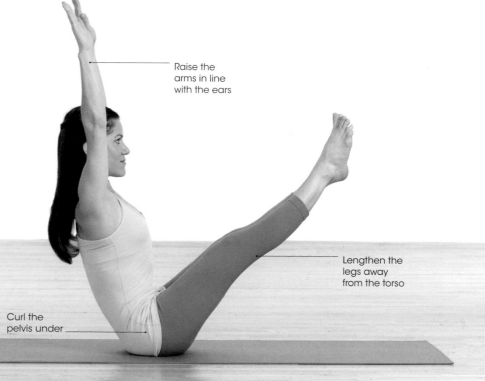

Raise the arms in line with the ears

Lengthen the legs away from the torso

Curl the pelvis under

4 Exhale and lower all the way down as slowly as possible, keeping your abs pulled in tightly. Lower your entire torso before your limbs touch down. Snap right back up in your letter "V" (Step 2) and repeat, descending more slowly each time.

HOW MANY DO I DO?
Perform 5 reps

TEMPO
Slow to moderate

Stretch away as you descend

Lower the body as much as possible

Keep the legs rotated in Pilates stance

Roll through one vertebra at a time

Rocking
Focus on control

In Pilates we often stretch, then counter-stretch. In Teaser III (see pp.190–91) you'll have been stretching your spine one way and in this Rocking exercise, you'll be stretching it the opposite way. Approach this move slowly to keep your balance.

1 Lie face down on your mat and bend your knees behind you to take hold of your ankles. Keep your legs parallel. Lift your head up and press your shoulders back.

Stretch the arms evenly back

Keep the knees close together

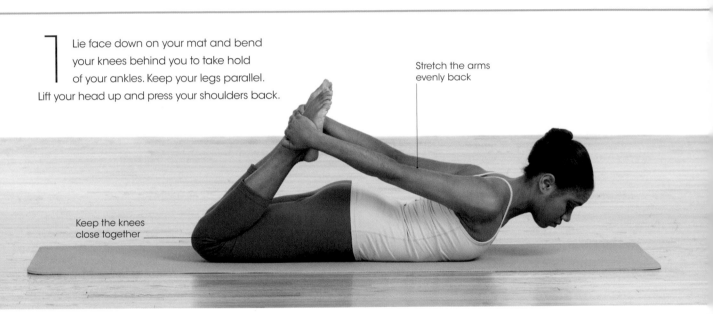

2 Looking straight ahead, gently stretch upwards by pressing your ankles back into your hands. Lift your chest high and find your balance. Lift your thighs up by pulling your feet higher.

Press the ankles into the hands

Keep the arms straight

3 Breathing naturally, begin a
small backward and forward
rocking motion. Each time you
rock, increase the range of motion
as much as possible. Release your
feet and sit on your heels to finish.

HOW MANY DO I DO?
Perform 6–10 reps

TEMPO
Moderate

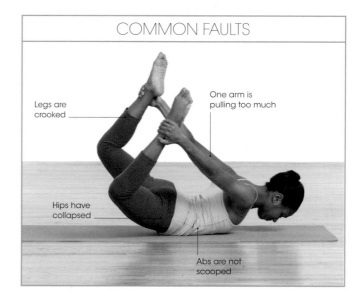

COMMON FAULTS

Legs are
crooked

One arm is
pulling too much

Hips have
collapsed

Abs are not
scooped

Keep the legs
parallel

Support the
abdominals

Leg Pull Down
Focus on precision

Front-supported planks are great for core strength. Leg Pull Down will build on that strength. This move involves you taking one leg up, which requires you to work that much harder. For the best results, focus on your mid-section rather than your limbs.

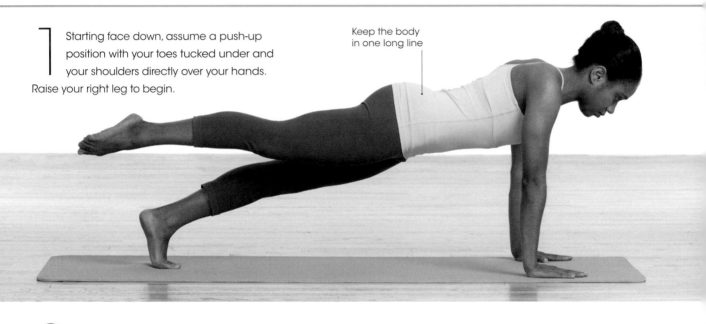

1 Starting face down, assume a push-up position with your toes tucked under and your shoulders directly over your hands. Raise your right leg to begin.

Keep the body in one long line

2 Breathing naturally throughout, press your left heel back and down with a double pulse. Keep your abs supported and your hips lifted.

Keep the hips level

Drop the heel

3 Shoot forward, rolling up on the ball of your left foot or higher. Replace your right foot next to your left. Raise your left leg to begin again. Continue alternating. Bend your knees to the mat to finish.

HOW MANY DO I DO?
Alternate for 6–8 sets

TEMPO
Moderate to rapid

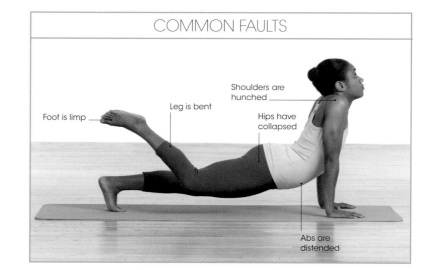

COMMON FAULTS

Foot is limp

Leg is bent

Shoulders are hunched

Hips have collapsed

Abs are distended

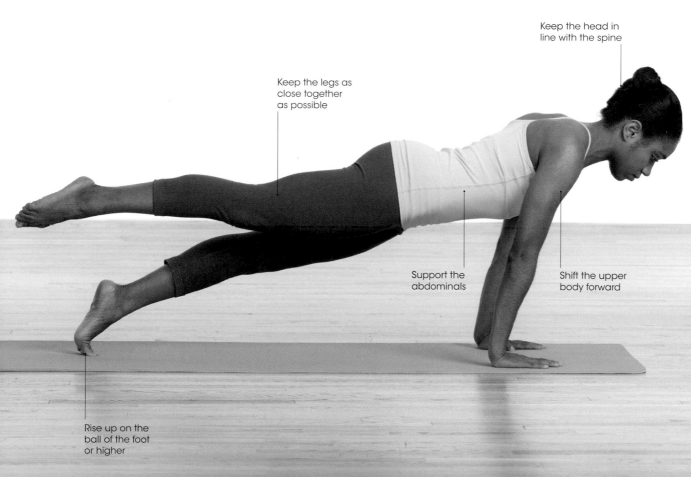

Keep the head in line with the spine

Keep the legs as close together as possible

Support the abdominals

Shift the upper body forward

Rise up on the ball of the foot or higher

Push-Ups
Focus on flow

Push-ups are so often avoided. These Pilates push-ups should never be left out.
Careful timing and precise form will rapidly improve your push-up technique.
Don't worry how many you can do – only how many perfect ones you can do.

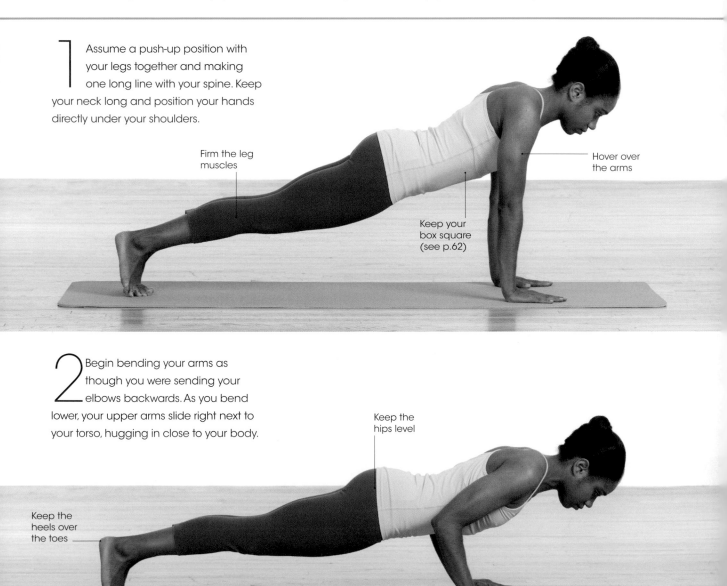

1 Assume a push-up position with your legs together and making one long line with your spine. Keep your neck long and position your hands directly under your shoulders.

Firm the leg muscles

Hover over the arms

Keep your box square (see p.62)

2 Begin bending your arms as though you were sending your elbows backwards. As you bend lower, your upper arms slide right next to your torso, hugging in close to your body.

Keep the hips level

Keep the heels over the toes

3 Continue lowering as far as you can for your level of strength. Take 3 full counts to lower. At your lowest point, your elbows should be above the level of your body. Hover for a moment, then push back up for 3 more counts. Repeat.

HOW MANY DO I DO?
Perform 3 reps

TEMPO
Moderate

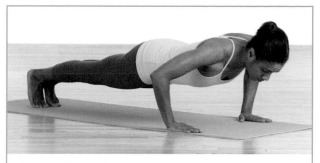

Too hard? Try this.
If you find holding the elbows in too challenging, allow them to open out to the sides until you are strong.

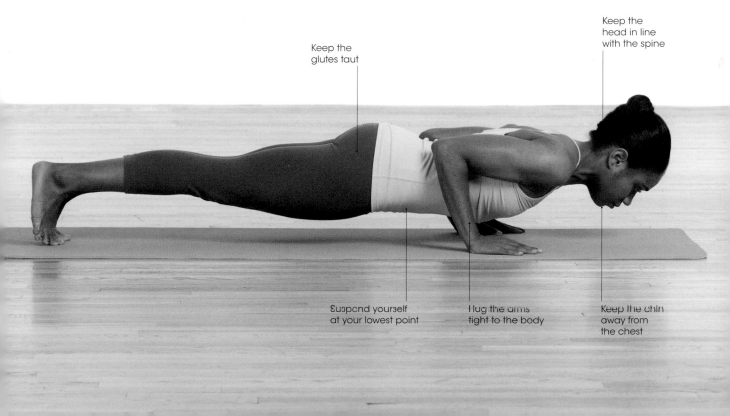

Keep the glutes taut

Keep the head in line with the spine

Suspend yourself at your lowest point

Hug the arms tight to the body

Keep the chin away from the chest

Kneeling Side Kicks
Focus on concentration

Side kicks become extremely challenging when you have to do them from an upright position. Working with a smaller base of support and farther off the ground requires even more core control. Kick each leg with rhythm and strength.

STARTING POSITION

Tighten the core

Take the knees just wider than the hips

1 Kneel upright on your mat, then drop down to the left, placing your left hand flat on the mat directly under your left shoulder. Take your right hand behind your head and point your elbow to the ceiling. Raise your right leg parallel to the floor and hold your torso strong and still.

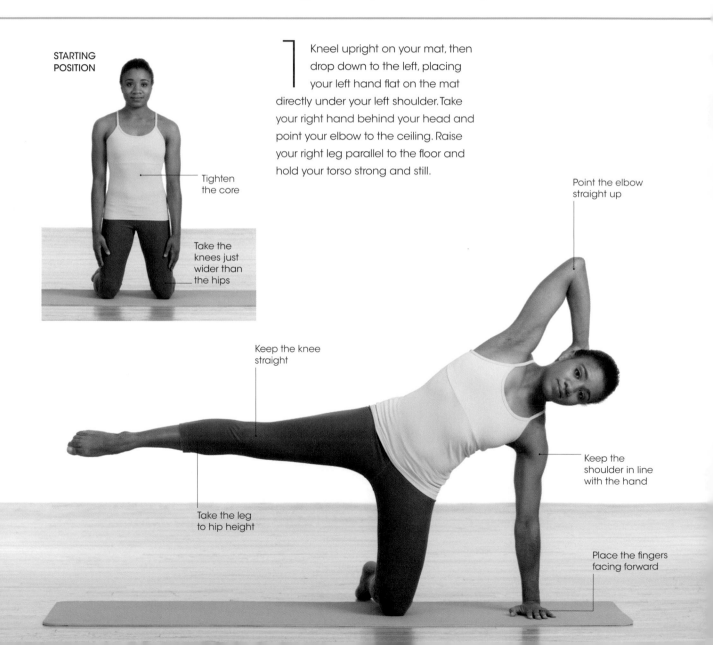

Point the elbow straight up

Keep the knee straight

Keep the shoulder in line with the hand

Take the leg to hip height

Place the fingers facing forward

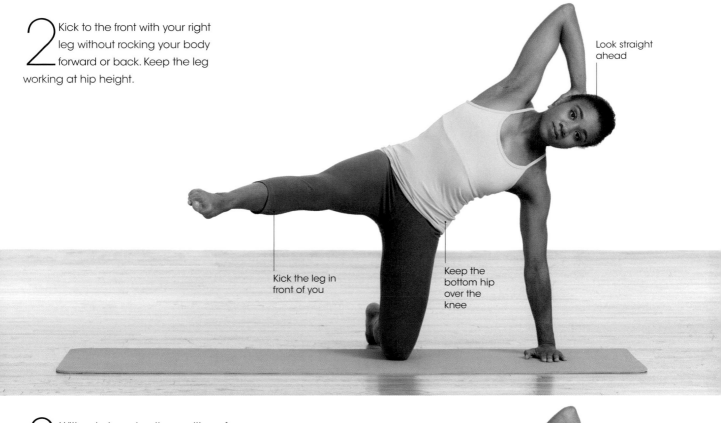

2 Kick to the front with your right leg without rocking your body forward or back. Keep the leg working at hip height.

Look straight ahead

Kick the leg in front of you

Keep the bottom hip over the knee

3 Without changing the position of your torso, kick your right leg back behind you. Repeat 5 times. To switch sides, push yourself off the mat and return to your upright kneeling position (Step 1, inset).

Keep the leg parallel to the floor

HOW MANY DO I DO?
Perform 5 reps, then switch sides for 5 reps

TEMPO
Moderate

Hold the arm strong as you swing back

Keep the back foot in line with the knee

Thigh Stretch
Focus on control

Don't let the name fool you. You will certainly get a stretch here, but this is a strengthening exercise. Work within your safe range of motion but be sure to focus on your progress. Each time you repeat the exercise, it should be better than the time before.

1 Kneel upright with your legs hip-width apart and a small weight in each hand. Raise your arms and reach them in front of you, just above hip height. Tighten your glutes, lower your chin and inhale to begin.

2 Exhale as you hinge back, keeping your body in a straight line from head to knees. Pause at your lowest point for a breath. Squeeze your buttock muscles tighter and spring back to upright with control. Repeat.

HOW MANY DO I DO?
Perform 5 reps

TEMPO
Slow

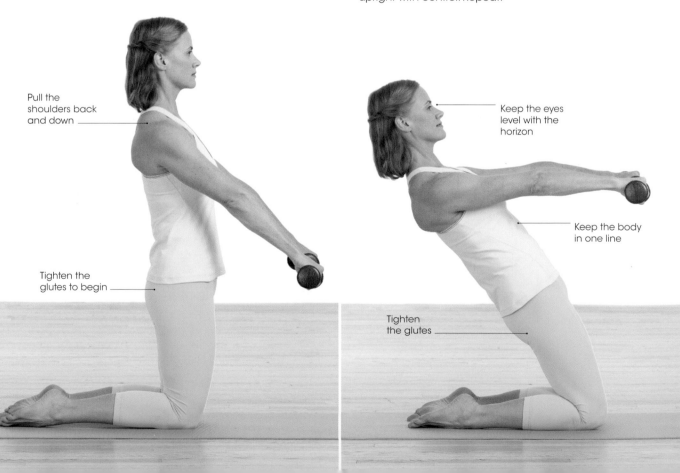

Pull the shoulders back and down

Tighten the glutes to begin

Keep the eyes level with the horizon

Keep the body in one line

Tighten the glutes

Side Bends
Focus on centring

Stillness is not one of the elements emphasised in Pilates. Rather than perform a static hold, we always expect the muscles to work hard in any given posture. Side Bends demonstrate this nicely with a small but difficult movement.

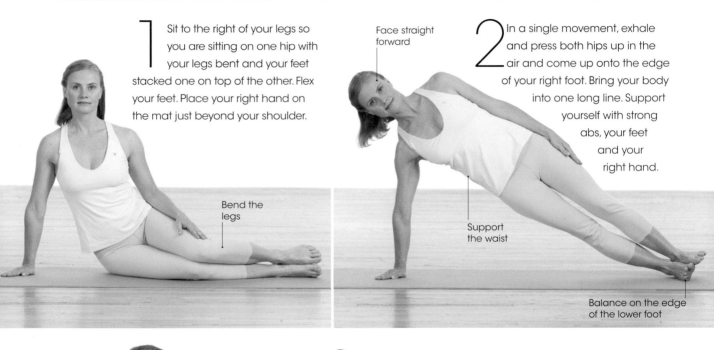

1 Sit to the right of your legs so you are sitting on one hip with your legs bent and your feet stacked one on top of the other. Flex your feet. Place your right hand on the mat just beyond your shoulder.

Bend the legs

2 In a single movement, exhale and press both hips up in the air and come up onto the edge of your right foot. Bring your body into one long line. Support yourself with strong abs, your feet and your right hand.

Face straight forward

Support the waist

Balance on the edge of the lower foot

Turn the head towards the legs

3 Dip your hips down towards the mat without bending your arms or legs. Look down along your legs. Try to touch the mat first with your bottom right calf, then with your right hip, before lifting up once more. Inhale as you lower, and exhale each time you lift.

Keep the legs stacked

HOW MANY DO I DO?
Perform 5 reps, then switch sides for 5 reps

TEMPO
Slow

Star
Focus on precision

Star is the ultimate type of side-plank. Once your Side Bends are proficient, Star will take your practice to the next level by testing your stability and strength both at the same time. As you perform this move, work carefully and with control.

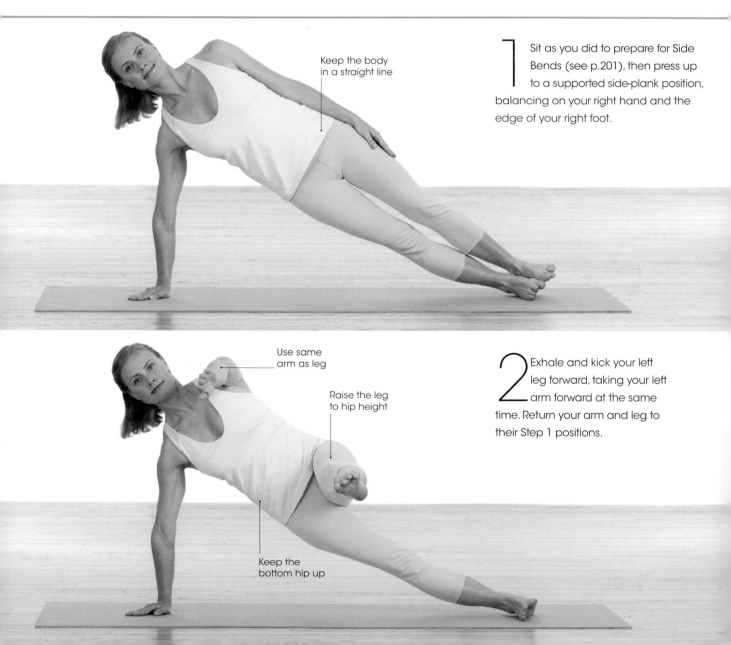

Keep the body
in a straight line

1 Sit as you did to prepare for Side Bends (see p.201), then press up to a supported side-plank position, balancing on your right hand and the edge of your right foot.

Use same
arm as leg

Raise the leg
to hip height

Keep the
bottom hip up

2 Exhale and kick your left leg forward, taking your left arm forward at the same time. Return your arm and leg to their Step 1 positions.

3 Now kick your left leg back and take your left arm forward. Lower them to begin again. Repeat, alternating front and back before lowering down onto your mat to switch sides.

HOW MANY DO I DO?
Perform 4–5 reps, then switch sides for 4–5 reps

TEMPO
Slow to moderate

Too hard? Try this.
If balancing on the edge of one foot is too hard, try placing one foot in front of the other. Hold this position until you feel steady enough to progress.

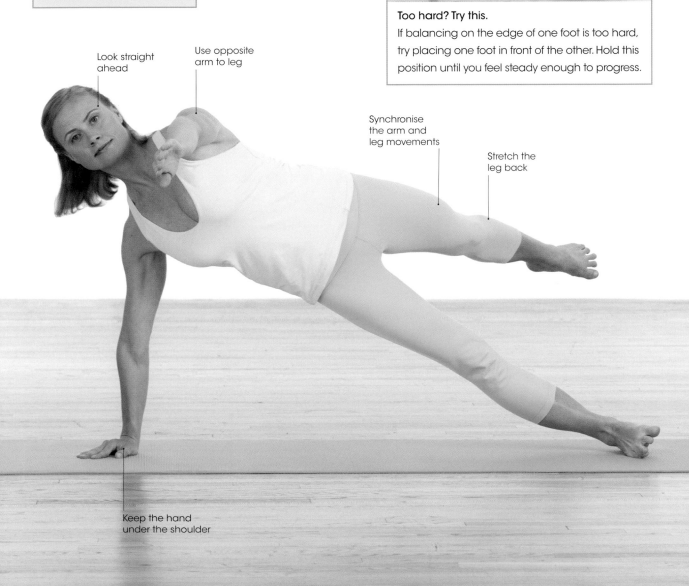

Look straight ahead

Use opposite arm to leg

Synchronise the arm and leg movements

Stretch the leg back

Keep the hand under the shoulder

Seal
Focus on flow

This final rolling exercise rounds off your Pilates programme. The Pilates approach is defined as minimum of effort for maximum efficiency. Intended to massage your spine and regulate your breathing, Seal should follow this rule.

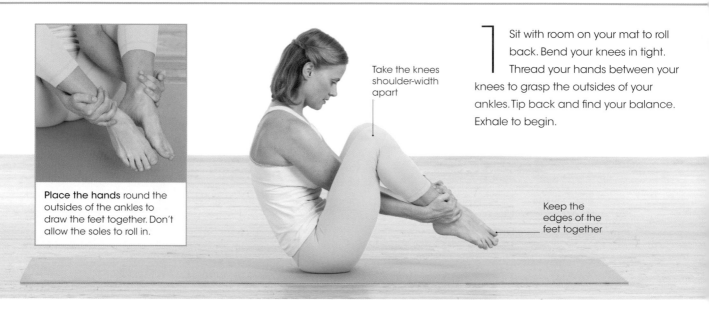

Place the hands round the outsides of the ankles to draw the feet together. Don't allow the soles to roll in.

Take the knees shoulder-width apart

Keep the edges of the feet together

1 Sit with room on your mat to roll back. Bend your knees in tight. Thread your hands between your knees to grasp the outsides of your ankles. Tip back and find your balance. Exhale to begin.

2 Inhale and roll back smoothly, allowing your hips to roll right up to the ceiling. Keep your head tucked in and off the mat. Hold your abs in as you roll.

3 Exhale as you roll forward, working your abs to roll back up to Step 1. Continue rolling back and forth, aiming your feet towards the mat but without letting them touch down.

HOW MANY DO I DO?
Perform 10 reps

TEMPO
Moderate

Keep the head off the floor

Coordinate your breath with your roll

Roll fluidly through the spine

Standing Swings
Focus on breath

There are videos of Mr Pilates on the internet that include moves which have never been formalised in any certification programme. Standing Swings is one of those. Remember that any Pilates workout should end upright to prepare you for your day.

1 Stand tall with your feet parallel, your legs hip-width apart and your arms long by your sides. Breathe in with the air and pull your abs in as you take your arms overhead, stretching up long and tall and slightly backwards.

Stretch up and back

Pull the waistline in and up

2 Exhale and drop down as if your upper body is falling. Let your knees bend deeply and your head drop down. Swing your arms through your legs and bounce your upper body 3 times at the lowest point. Inhale and swing up again to repeat.

HOW MANY DO I DO?
Perform 5–8 reps

TEMPO
Moderate to rapid

Stretch the arms through the legs

Standing Jumps
Focus on flow

I believe that all Pilates workouts should make you out of breath at least twice during your workout, if not more. Standing Jumps accomplishes this to a tee. It takes practice to jump well, so focus on your landings each time you perform this exercise.

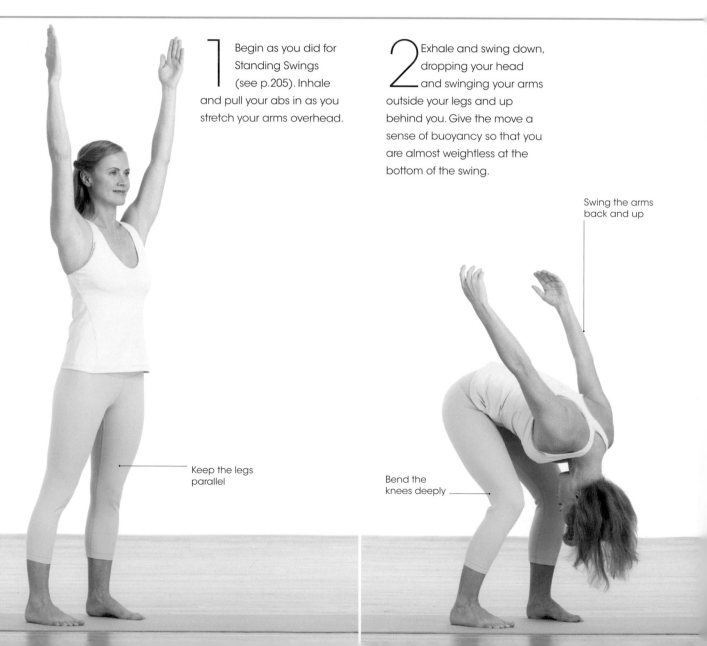

1 Begin as you did for Standing Swings (see p.205). Inhale and pull your abs in as you stretch your arms overhead.

2 Exhale and swing down, dropping your head and swinging your arms outside your legs and up behind you. Give the move a sense of buoyancy so that you are almost weightless at the bottom of the swing.

Swing the arms back and up

Keep the legs parallel

Bend the knees deeply

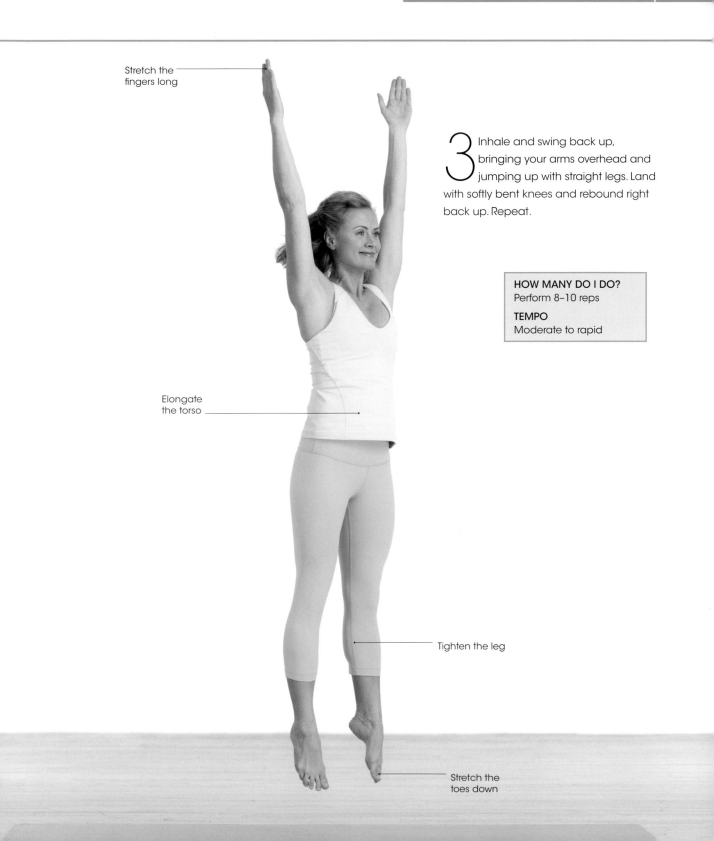

Stretch the fingers long

3 Inhale and swing back up, bringing your arms overhead and jumping up with straight legs. Land with softly bent knees and rebound right back up. Repeat.

HOW MANY DO I DO?
Perform 8–10 reps

TEMPO
Moderate to rapid

Elongate the torso

Tighten the leg

Stretch the toes down

15-minute sequence

Congratulations on making it to the Advanced sequence. Remember that advanced material does not mean you are an advanced student. All students are beginners. That's why we call it a "practice", so you can continue to do just that – practise.

1 The Hundred p.154
Perform 10 inhalations and
10 exhalations (100 pumps)
Stay on your back for no 2

2 Hip-Ups p.155
Perform 6 reps, pause
briefly, then perform 6
more reps
Sit up tall for no 3

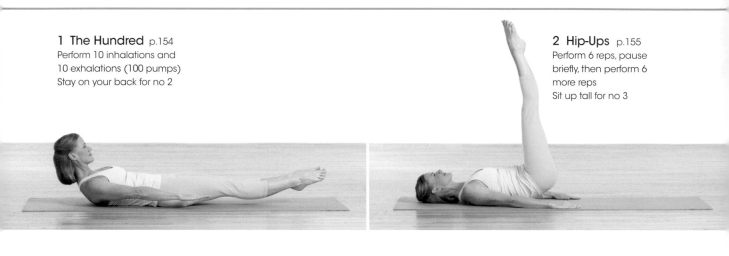

**3 Rolling Like
a Ball III** pp.160–61
Perform 8–10 reps
Lie back on your mat
for no 4

4 Footwork p.162
Perform 10 reps
Stay on your back for no 5

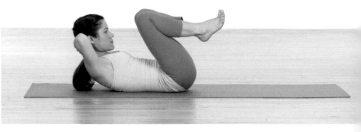

**5 Double
Straight Leg
Stretch** p.163
Perform 5–8 reps
Sit up straight for no 6

6 Spine Stretch Forward III
p.165
Perform 5 reps
Stay seated for no 7

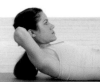

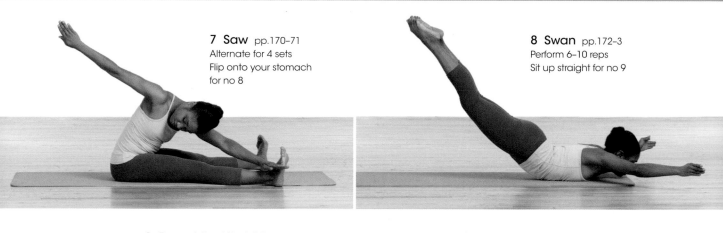

7 Saw pp.170–71
Alternate for 4 sets
Flip onto your stomach
for no 8

8 Swan pp.172–3
Perform 6–10 reps
Sit up straight for no 9

9 Round the World II pp.176–7
Alternate for 3 sets
Roll onto your left side for no 10

10 Side Kicks: Rond de Jambe pp.188–9
Perform 3 reps, then reverse direction for 3 reps,
then repeat on your right side
Come onto your knees for no 11

11 Thigh Stretch
p.200
Perform 5 reps
Sit towards the front of
your mat for no 12

**13 Standing
Swings** p.205
Perform 5–8 reps

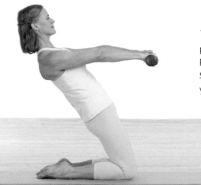

12 Seal p.204
Perform 10 reps
Come up to
standing for no 13

30-minute sequence

Welcome to the eighth programme in this book. You are almost at the finish line. Take a moment to reread the Benefits of Pilates and the Before you begin chapters before starting on this programme. Take a renewed interest in the foundations of Pilates.

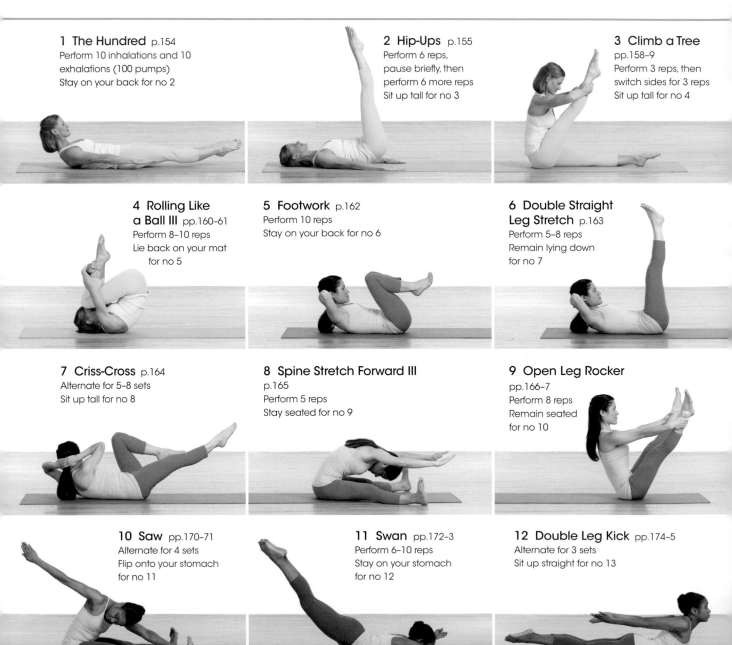

1 The Hundred p.154
Perform 10 inhalations and 10 exhalations (100 pumps)
Stay on your back for no 2

2 Hip-Ups p.155
Perform 6 reps, pause briefly, then perform 6 more reps
Sit up tall for no 3

3 Climb a Tree pp.158–9
Perform 3 reps, then switch sides for 3 reps
Sit up tall for no 4

4 Rolling Like a Ball III pp.160–61
Perform 8–10 reps
Lie back on your mat for no 5

5 Footwork p.162
Perform 10 reps
Stay on your back for no 6

6 Double Straight Leg Stretch p.163
Perform 5–8 reps
Remain lying down for no 7

7 Criss-Cross p.164
Alternate for 5–8 sets
Sit up tall for no 8

8 Spine Stretch Forward III p.165
Perform 5 reps
Stay seated for no 9

9 Open Leg Rocker pp.166–7
Perform 8 reps
Remain seated for no 10

10 Saw pp.170–71
Alternate for 4 sets
Flip onto your stomach for no 11

11 Swan pp.172–3
Perform 6–10 reps
Stay on your stomach for no 12

12 Double Leg Kick pp.174–5
Alternate for 3 sets
Sit up straight for no 13

13 Round the World II
pp.176–7
Alternate for 3 sets
Remain seated for no 14

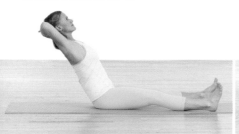

14 Spine Twist II pp.180–81
Alternate for 5 sets
Stay seated for no 15

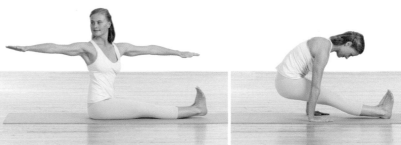

15 Tendon Stretch pp.182–3
Perform 5 reps
Roll onto your left side for no 16

16 Side Kicks: Bicycle pp.186–7
Perform 6 reps
Stay on your left side for no 17

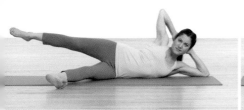

17 Side Kicks: Rond de Jambe
pp.188–9
Perform 3 reps, then reverse direction for 3 reps,
then repeat numbers 16 and 17 on your right side
Turn face down on the mat for no 18

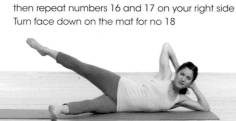

18 Leg Pull Down
pp.194–5
Alternate for 6–8 sets
Stay face down for no 19

19 Push-Ups pp.196–7
Perform 3 reps
Kneel sideways on the mat
for no 20

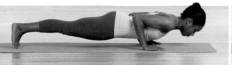

20 Kneeling Side Kicks pp.198–9
Perform 5 reps, then switch sides
for 5 reps
Pivot to face the front
of the mat for no 21

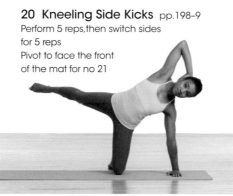

21 Thigh Stretch p.200
Perform 5 reps
Sit on your right hip for no 22

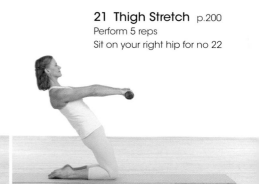

22 Side Bends p.201
Perform 5 reps, then switch
sides for 5 reps
Sit on your mat for no 23

23 Seal p.204
Perform 10 reps
Come up to standing for no 24

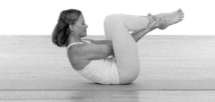

24 Standing Swings p.205
Perform 5–8 reps

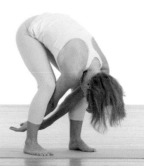

45-minute sequence

This is your final programme and will synthesise everything you have learned. It's tempting to throw caution to the wind as you pick up your tempo. Feel free to move swiftly but every now and then try a slower workout to keep your technique clean and solid.

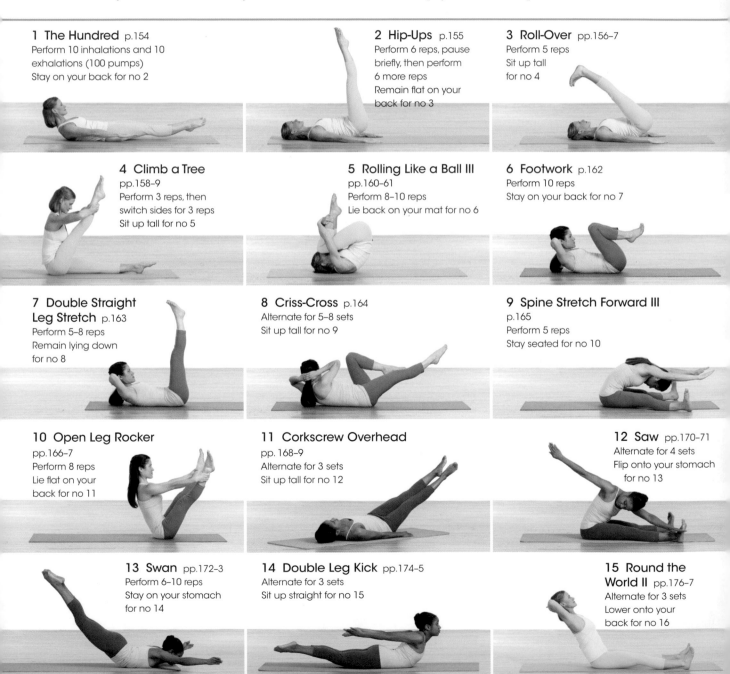

1 The Hundred p.154
Perform 10 inhalations and 10 exhalations (100 pumps)
Stay on your back for no 2

2 Hip-Ups p.155
Perform 6 reps, pause briefly, then perform 6 more reps
Remain flat on your back for no 3

3 Roll-Over pp.156-7
Perform 5 reps
Sit up tall for no 4

4 Climb a Tree pp.158-9
Perform 3 reps, then switch sides for 3 reps
Sit up tall for no 5

5 Rolling Like a Ball III pp.160-61
Perform 8-10 reps
Lie back on your mat for no 6

6 Footwork p.162
Perform 10 reps
Stay on your back for no 7

7 Double Straight Leg Stretch p.163
Perform 5-8 reps
Remain lying down for no 8

8 Criss-Cross p.164
Alternate for 5-8 sets
Sit up tall for no 9

9 Spine Stretch Forward III p.165
Perform 5 reps
Stay seated for no 10

10 Open Leg Rocker pp.166-7
Perform 8 reps
Lie flat on your back for no 11

11 Corkscrew Overhead pp.168-9
Alternate for 3 sets
Sit up tall for no 12

12 Saw pp.170-71
Alternate for 4 sets
Flip onto your stomach for no 13

13 Swan pp.172-3
Perform 6-10 reps
Stay on your stomach for no 14

14 Double Leg Kick pp.174-5
Alternate for 3 sets
Sit up straight for no 15

15 Round the World II pp.176-7
Alternate for 3 sets
Lower onto your back for no 16

16 Scissors
pp.178–9
Alternate for 5 sets
Sit up tall for no 17

17 Spine Twist II pp.180–81
Alternate for 5 sets
Stay seated for
no 18

18 Tendon Stretch pp.182–3
Perform 5 reps
Lower onto your back for no 19

19 Jackknife
pp.184–5
Perform 5 reps
Flip onto your left side
for no 20

20 Side Kicks: Bicycle pp.186–7
Perform 6 reps
Stay on your left side for no 21

21 Side Kicks: Rond de Jambe
pp.188–9
Perform 3 reps, then reverse direction for 3 reps,
then change sides and repeat numbers 20
and 21 on your right side
Roll onto your back for no 22

22 Teaser III pp.190–91
Perform 5 reps
Flip onto your stomach
for no 23

23 Rocking pp.192–3
Perform 6–10 reps
Stay face down
for no 24

24 Leg Pull Down
pp.194–5
Alternate for 6–8 sets
Stay face down for no 25

25 Push-Ups pp.196–7
Perform 3 reps
Kneel sideways on the mat
for no 26

26 Kneeling Side Kicks
pp.198–9
Perform 5 reps,
then switch
sides for 5 reps
Pivot to face the front
of the mat for no 27

**27 Thigh
Stretch** p.200
Perform 5 reps
Sit on your right
hip for no 28

28 Side Bends p.201
Perform 5 reps, then switch
sides for 5 reps
Stay on your side for no 29

29 Star
pp.202–3
Perform 4–5 reps, then switch
sides for 4–5 reps
Sit on your mat for no 30

30 Seal p.204
Perform 10 reps
Come up to
standing for no 31

**31 Standing
Swings** p.205
Perform 5–8 reps
Remain standing
for no 32

**32
Standing
Jumps**
pp.206–7
Perform
8–10 reps

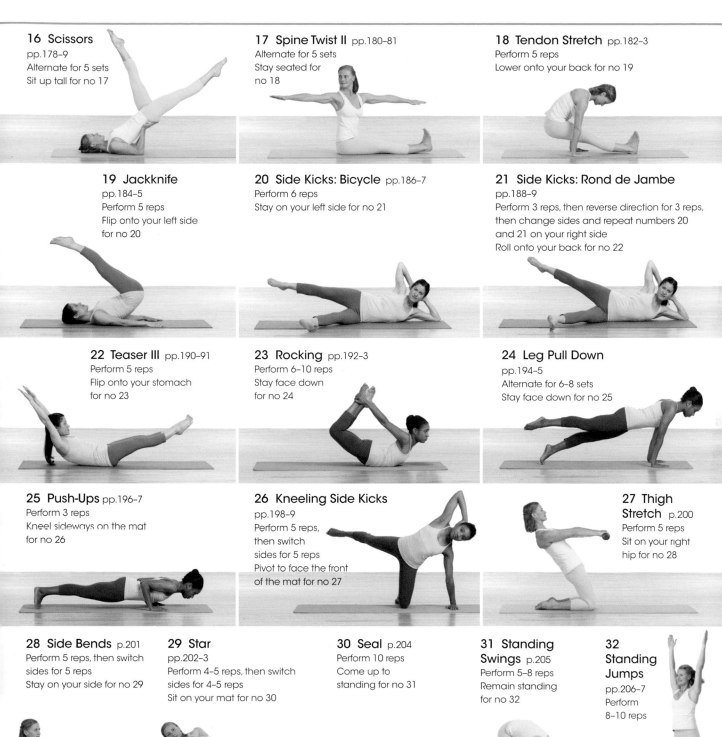
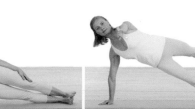

Troubleshooting

Pilates is tough. The challenges are unique and the method gets harder the more you practise. Although I want desperately to hold your hand through your training, it just isn't possible. However, I am able to predict some of the most common barriers and give you a few simple suggestions and possible solutions.

Pilates problem solving

There will be exercises you meet along your Pilates path that will confound and frustrate you. How do you know when to proceed and when to find an alternative? Follow these guidelines to help you map out your own success strategy. Let's work our way backwards from exercises you might eliminate or substitute to moves you will modify.

ELIMINATION

If you have a condition or injury that prevents you from doing certain movements, simply leave them out. Skipping over a movement is often safer than trying to adjust it to fit your needs. For example, if a spinal problem prevents you from performing rolling exercises, omit the movement and progress to the next exercise. When you're stronger, revisit the exercise.

SUBSTITUTION

If you find yourself unable to do a certain exercise but are able to complete other similar moves, substitution is a good option. If we stick with the example of rolling, many people can perform Seal (see p.204) but can't execute Rolling Like a Ball III (see p.160). Is it OK to substitute? In a word, yes. The only caveat is – don't give up. Your goal is to successfully complete every exercise in this book, so continue to work hard at each and every move.

MODIFICATION

If you can do some of an exercise but not all of it, make a change to the move. I usually recommend performing just a portion of it. There's no need to change the steps or reorganise the choreography; just abbreviate the exercise so that you can accomplish some part of it. If you can't come all the way up from Rolling Like a Ball, don't. Just rock back and forth at the bottom-most portion of the move, gradually gaining strength and mobility until one day – presto! You'll find that you float right up to the top. I guarantee this strategy works with every exercise.

What if I can't?

There's a way to work round the problem for every possible movement limitation you might have. Here are my no-nonsense answers to many of the common issues that arise during the process of Pilates training.

Q *What if I can't do a sit-up?*
A Sit-ups usually involve lying flat and coming fully upright. Thankfully, in this book, you'll do very little of that. I have reorganised most of the sit-up-style moves to work from the top down. Instead of sitting up from lying down, you'll sit up and lower yourself down. Go as far as you can each time.

Q *What if I can't arch my back upwards?*
A Not being able to bend backwards or arch upwards from a face-down position is usually the result of too little mobility along the spine. Spend some time on your stomach every day. Up to two minutes at a time, lie face down propped up on your arms and allow your spine to bend in a relaxed position. This may be uncomfortable at first, but in time, your mobility will increase.

Q *What if I can't keep my legs straight?*
A Tight muscles resist lengthening in many moves. It's OK to allow your legs to bend as long as you continually exert effort to straighten them. With practice, your muscles will lengthen and it will become much easier.

Q *What if it's not hard enough?*
A No such thing. You may not be working hard enough. Or possibly you are speeding through the hard parts of each exercise. Focus on the moves that are difficult for you. Slow down and work harder.

Q *What if I'm stuck on an exercise?*
A Keep trying it. Still stuck? Break it apart into little sections and work out which piece is troubling you. Practise that small piece relentlessly.

Q *What if I just can't remember the order of the routine?*
A You can't escape good old-fashioned memorisation. Use a catchy tune or mnemonic to help you remember your list of exercises. You must commit it to memory. Just get it done.

BOTTOM LINE
I can give you all the rules, guidelines and suggestions in the world but you'll do best to follow your instincts. Learn to listen to your body when it needs to stop or make a change. Be consistent and committed.

The perfect workout

Working out what's hard and what's easy is the key to customising your workout. Take time to assess each move and your own ability to create your perfect routine.

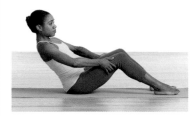

IT'S TOO EASY
If an exercise feels too easy, you probably aren't doing it right.

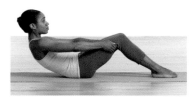

IT'S TOO HARD
If it's too hard, you're on the right track. Keep practising, but modify if needed.

Joining a class

If you're considering joining a class, go right ahead and jump in. Working out at home is always an option but there's no substitute for live instruction. Even occasional classes are sure to amplify the workouts you do on your own.

Pilates teachers and classes come in all shapes and sizes. Some fast, some slow. Some classical, some contemporary. Some have music, some have props. There are no rules that distinguish a good class from a bad class. I define the "best" class as the one you'll return to over and over again.

Group classes are usually structured in a straightforward manner. Students gather on mats and are taken through a Pilates routine for up to an hour at a time. The focus of the class is the teacher's voice. Most Pilates teachers perform some type of manual adjustments to their students, so you may find yourself being stretched or manipulated at some point.

When it's over, you should feel that you have had a full-body workout. A sense of fatigue is normal but you should also feel invigorated.

Before you can set about finding a class, you need to be clear about your own goals. Why are you going to Pilates class? What do you want to achieve? Answer these questions for yourself and you'll be ready to begin your hunt for the perfect class.

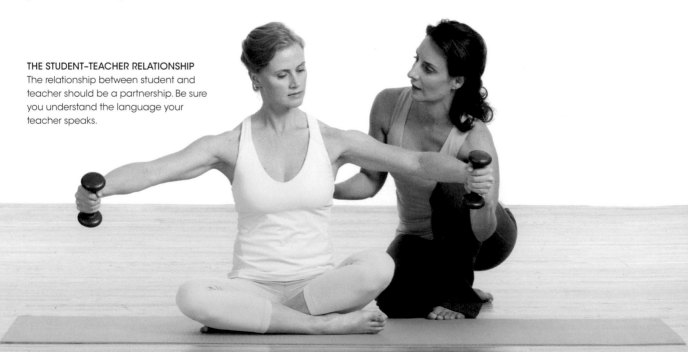

THE STUDENT–TEACHER RELATIONSHIP
The relationship between student and teacher should be a partnership. Be sure you understand the language your teacher speaks.

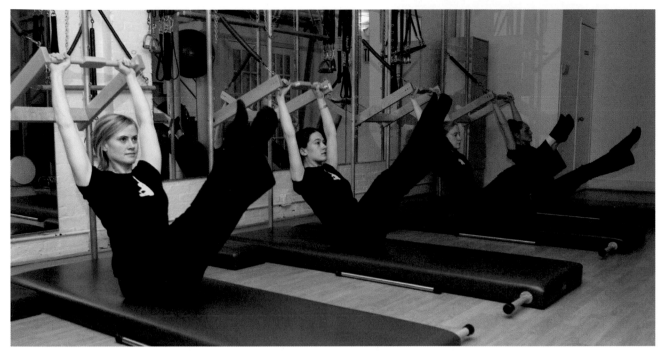

GROUP CLASSES COME IN ALL GUISES
Some studios offer only Pilates mat work, while others utilise various equipment. Try as many styles as you can.

Finding the right teacher

To find the most suitable teacher, let's recall your primary school for a moment. Do you remember your favourite teacher? There's usually one who stood out, who helped you understand a topic you struggled with. Someone you really connected with. That's the type of rapport you want to have with your Pilates teacher. Communication is key to your success.

Here are some tips to help you make the best possible choice. First, do your homework. Ask your friends and family who they know and who they would recommend for you. If you draw a blank, check your local bodywork practitioners. Massage therapists, yoga teachers and even spas and salons should be able to point you in the right direction.

Armed with a few referrals, the next step is to phone any prospective teachers to find out what they are offering. Ask about their style of training and their experience and share your particular goals with them. Any trainer worth their salt will ask you what you are hoping to achieve with Pilates so that they can assess your compatibility.

Many new teachers are experienced in other therapies, so you shouldn't write someone off just because they're new. Finally, if at all possible, go and observe a class. It's quite likely that out of every five classes you try, three will be just fine. One will be a terrible match and one will be extraordinary. Hold out for the extraordinary. Shop around for the best training you can get.

Assessing the class

You'll know straight away if the class was right for you. Did you feel energised and satisfied with the workout? If so, great. If not, it may warrant another visit before you try another class.

Do be aware of what I call "red flags", which signal that this isn't a class you want to repeat.

• The teacher doesn't greet you, ask your name or ask if there are any conditions they should be aware of.

• You have localised pain that doesn't go away in a few days after the class.

• You aren't sore at all after the class.

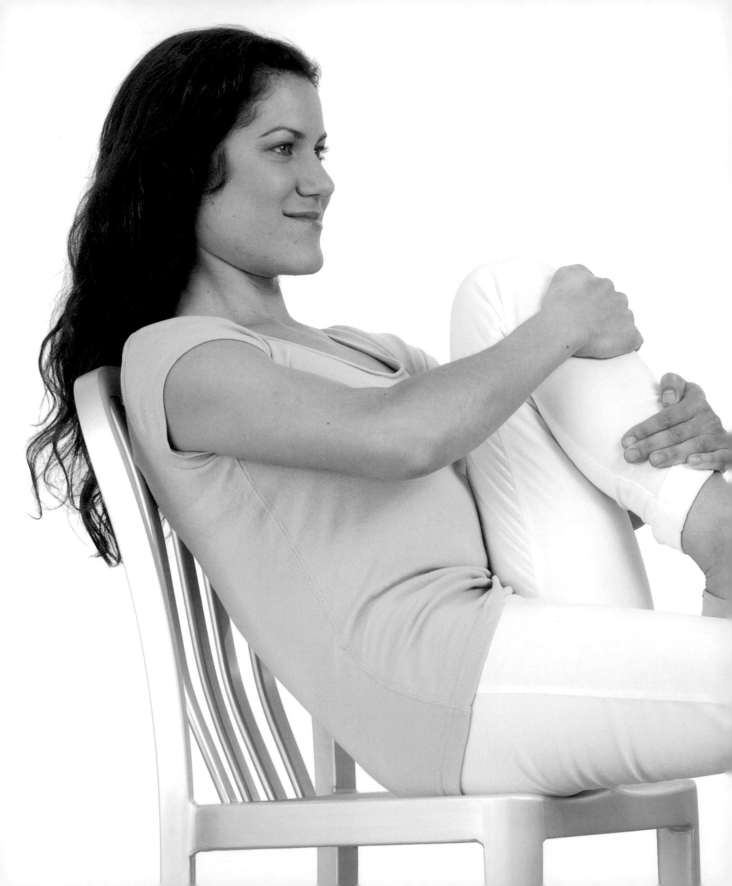

Pilates
Every Day

From workout to daily life

Pilates should become a way of life for you. The principles and ideals are easily manifest in your daily living. I don't mean to suggest that you should burst into exercise at family functions, but the way you hold your body during your workout should be reflected each and every day in your day-to-day activities. There are many opportunities to use your Pilates in your daily life.

It may not seem that simply lying on a mat and making certain shapes with your body would have a profound effect on your daily performance. But Pilates really is more than just exercise. It's a complete reprogramming of bad habits and the implementation of healthy biomechanical patterns. You can expect to see the following elements of Pilates become pervasive in every area of your life:

- The principles of proper breathing (see p.46) stay with you all day long.
- The principles of control and concentration (see p.42) seep into your other activities and into your work.
- The concept of centring (see p.44) begins to be second nature when you're engaged in other physical activities.

Pilates is the only exercise routine I know of that you can take right outside the door with you from your very first workout.

To help you customise your workout for your specific needs in your real life, you'll find a Know your body section on pages 222–3. Use this spread to help you develop your own personal workout plan for the short and long term.

Pilates for real life

The remainder of this chapter includes a variety of short workouts that you can use to supplement your existing workouts. In these short workouts, you'll learn how Pilates has particular applications in the elderly (see pp.236–9), in rehabilitation (see pp.240–43) and for sport and play (see pp.226–7). I've also included workouts for you to do at your office (see pp.228–9) and a workout that will definitely improve your sex life (see pp.232–5). Finally, I've written a diet section (see pp.244–9). This should start you on your way to overall fitness and wellness.

"Through Contrology you first purposefully acquire complete control of your own body and then through proper repetition of its exercises, you gradually and progressively acquire that natural rhythm and coordination associated with all your subconscious activities." Joseph Pilates

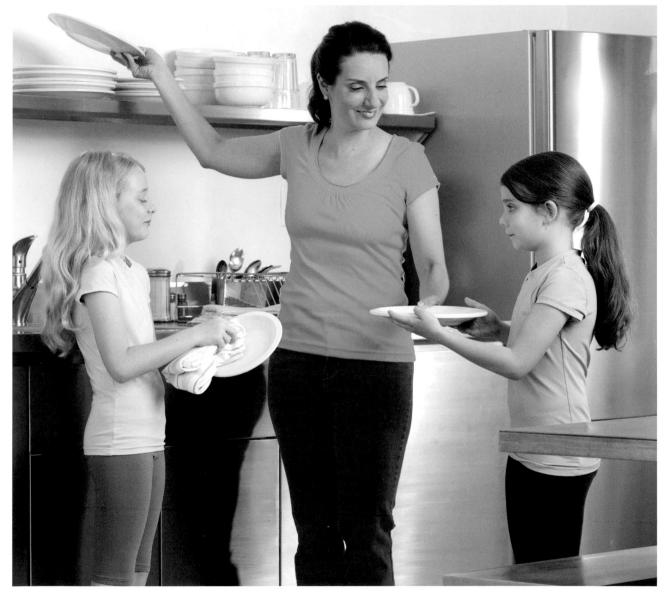

A WAY OF LIFE
Your workout should help your life. Pilates makes family activities that much easier by training you to carry your body efficiently. When you stand tall, so does everyone else.

Be the change

We're more sedentary than ever and our children are virtually shackled to one type of screen or another all day. We're their role models, so we must influence them to take better care of their bodies from the start. Kids are naturally physical. If they see you doing Pilates, they'll naturally engage. Similarly, if you talk about health and fitness, they'll absorb the message.

Remember that, over time, Pilates isn't just something you do. It becomes something you are. And by inspiring others, you can really make a difference.

Know your body

If you're just learning Pilates, your body will need time to absorb this new way of moving and you'll almost certainly feel muscles you haven't felt before. You may be sore in places you're unfamiliar with. Exercises that seem easy at first glance may be far more difficult than you imagined.

The following general guidelines don't apply for all conditions, but I've had great success recommending these adjustments for specific limitations.

Your Pilates prescription

BAD KNEE?
Avoid bending too tight or straightening too hard. If you're pulling a knee towards your chest, adjust to hold behind the thigh rather than on top of the knee or shin. When lengthening your leg, avoid hyperextending or "locking out" the knee. Focus on strengthening your quads and hamstrings equally.

DELICATE NECK?
Avoid neck strain by working abdominal moves in reverse. Start from a sitting-up position and go back instead of starting low and lifting. Improve your neck alignment with exercises like Wall: Stand (see p.96) and Neck Presses (see p.64).

WEAK HIP?
Focus on strengthening your legs and gluteals. Exercises like Bottom Walk (see pp.80–81), Mini Bridge (see p.115) and Leg Swings: Side (see p.144) will help accomplish this, as well as the entire Side Kicks series (see pp.85–7, 130–33 and 186–9).

WEAK SHOULDER?
Keep the arm working safely within the joint and avoid extreme motion such as stretching the arm too far out or back. Work to strengthen the shoulder with moves like Side Bends (see p.201) and Sparklers (see p.95).

DELICATE WRIST?
Work on strength and alignment. Modify moves like Push-Ups (see pp.196–7) and Tendon Stretch (see pp.182–3) by supporting yourself on your fists.

Practise keeping long wrists during moves like Front Curls (see p.93) and Chest Expansion (see p.102).

WEAK SPINE?

All backs need strengthening regardless of their history or condition. Swan Prep (see p.83), Knee Stretches (see p.84) and Swimming (see p.138) are good places to start.

BAD ANKLE?

For sensitive ankles, make use of the Two by Four (see p.99) exercise to reinforce good alignment. You may also use Foot Walk (see p.238) from the Maturing with Pilates section to strengthen the smaller muscles of the feet.

Your own Pilates plan

You learned in the beginning of the book how to set some short-term goals (see p.41). It's now time to attend to your long-term goals. Let's use an imaginary student to demonstrate how you would build a chart for your personal Pilates plan.

John started Pilates 10 weeks ago. His goals were to improve his breathing, increase his flexibility and build stamina. After charting his original baseline measurements (see p.17), he began practising the Beginner programme three times a week. He plotted troublesome exercises into his chart, categorising each in either the breathing column or the flexibility column. He also included a note about which part was difficult for each move.

After six weeks, he recorded new measurements to compare with his original findings. Finally, he noted whatever improvements he had made in the individual exercises. His data is presented **in bold** for your easy reference. Create a chart like this for yourself, using your own goals to help you visualise your workouts and your results. Real Pilates is all about knowing your body and making the best possible gains. Use the tools in this book to become your own coach and guide. By so doing, you can achieve any goal you set.

GOALS	BASELINE	CHALLENGE MOVES	BASELINE 6 WEEK RE-TEST	CHALLENGE MOVES 6 WEEK RE-TEST
Improve breath capacity	Breathing – can manage a 5-second exhalation	Hundred Prep – only able to do one set of 40	Breathing – can manage a 12-second exhalation!	Hundred Prep – able to do one set of 50 and a second set of 25
Alignment	–			
Strength	–			
Stability	–			
Become more flexible	Flexibility – can only Leg Raise to 130° and with knee bent	Single Leg Circles – can't keep legs straight or get leg up to ceiling	Straight Leg Raise – can now manage 110°, and much straighter!	Single Leg Circles – bottom leg straight now. This feels much easier
Body control	–			
Body shape and tone	–			
Build stamina	Endurance – Wall: Chair – can hold for 20 seconds	Footwork – can only do 5 reps Swimming – can do 8–10 sets	Wall: Chair – can hold up to 40 seconds	Footwork – can do up to 10 reps! Swimming – can do up to 15 sets!
Mind over muscle	–			
Stress reduction	–			

Maintaining good posture

Pilates posture is distinctive. You can see it the minute someone walks in the room. Posture, in and of itself, is something we consider from a static perspective. But a Pilates-trained body demonstrates good posture dynamically, with every movement. With regular Pilates training, you will improve your posture significantly.

The human body is designed for mobility. Our skeletal support structure is a collection of hundreds of bones joined together to provide us with maximum mobility and a modicum of stability. Sitting or standing for a lengthy period is not what we were designed to do.

Getting good posture isn't difficult. Maintaining good posture is. You won't be able to overhaul your posture in a day or even a week. But as your Pilates practice develops, you'll discover that your poor postural habits become increasingly uncomfortable. You'll find yourself regularly adjusting, fidgeting and making other small movements to improve your stance.

You should dispel the notion that good posture means stiffening or freezing your spine. The ideal posture is a dynamic alignment

EXAMPLE OF POOR SITTING POSTURE
The trunk is collapsed and the shoulders are rolled forward. The back of the neck is shortened and the spine is rounded and hunched.

EXAMPLE OF GOOD SITTING POSTURE
Here, the weight is shifted slightly forward in the chair, bringing more weight onto the feet and allowing the lower back to assume a more natural curve. The shoulders and neck all fall into good alignment.

that cleverly adapts for changes in position, balance and pressure all day long by making almost imperceptible calibrations.

WHILE QUEUING Standing in a queue taking its toll on your tall, long posture? Try shifting your weight to one side, bending one foot up behind you but trying to keep your hips level. Keep shifting in 10-second increments. You may also consider squatting. Many cultures utilise the squat routinely. If you aren't in the habit of squatting, try practising at home. It's great for mobility and the digestive system and also provides a respite for lengthy standing.

WHILE WORKING Hunched over your keyboard? Sitting back in your chair is a fine strategy but try rolling a small towel up to place behind your lower back. This can help alleviate lower-back pain. As an alternative, sit towards the front edge of your chair with your feet firmly on the floor. Some people find a small wedge under the glutes helps avoid back strain. Be sure to leave your seat or take an overhead stretch at least once every 15 to 30 minutes.

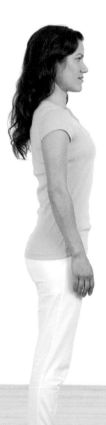
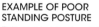

EXAMPLE OF POOR STANDING POSTURE
This one-legged weight-shift is causing the hips to be uneven and the spine to be misaligned. The upper body leans and twists to compensate for the imbalance in the lower body.

EXAMPLE OF GOOD STANDING POSTURE
In this example, the weight is evenly distributed through the lower limbs. The skeleton is neatly stacked, with the upper body directly over the lower body. The arms hang loose and the neck is well aligned.

Pilates for sport and play

I've already remarked that I consider Pilates to be cross-training for real life. People who do Pilates do more of everything else. They use Pilates to train their bodies to excel at real life, and sport and play are part of that.

Pilates makes you comfortable and confident as you move. When you feel at ease moving, you're more likely to participate in sport and play. If you're already athletic, Pilates can enhance your sports-specific abilities. Individual sports participants like skiers, skaters and runners or swimmers benefit tremendously from Pilates' focus and concentration (see p.42).

CRISS-CROSS (see p.164)
The abdominal oblique muscles help your body rotate and twist. Use this exercise to strengthen those movements as well as increase your coordination and range of motion.
Good for? Tennis, golf, boxing and baseball.

Focus on a stronger twist to each side, increasing the twist each time

MINI BRIDGE (see p.114)
The gluteal and hamstring (back-of-thigh) muscles are important for power moves and overall lower-body strength. Use this exercise to increase your ability to jump and stretch as well as develop your stamina.
Good for? Volleyball and basketball.

Focus on sustaining your position, pressing up higher each time

The integration of mind and muscle (see pp.34–5) is especially ideal for the execution of sports you do alone. By practising Pilates and honing your attention to detail (see p.45) and coordination of movement, you'll see a marked improvement in your sports performance.

Lovers of team sports, who participate in activities like football, volleyball and basketball, will be able to improve their timing, balance and flexibility (see pp.26–9). Pilates training will virtually guarantee a reduction in sports-related injuries as well as an improvement in recovery time.

Playtime as a pastime is vital for emotional and mental wellbeing. The ability to roll around with your children, chase a Frisbee with a pet or play tag with your friends is something many of us opt out of when given the chance. The practice of Pilates is playful. Rolling exercises and animal names combined with strength and conditioning movements make for a lighthearted yet effective workout. Pilates will help you play harder and better.

SIDE BENDS (see p.201)
Muscles along the side of the body lend extra stability to your torso and hips. Use the Side Bends to increase the strength and mobility of your waist.
Good for? Skiing, football and running.

Focus on bending more deeply each time

LEG PULL DOWN (see pp.194–5)
Deep abdominal muscles can never get too much strength. Use the Leg Pull Down to improve your core stabilisation and increase your upper-body strength, as well as promote better alignment.
Good for? Swimming and cycling.

Focus on a strong centre, pulling the abs tighter each time

Pilates at the office

It goes without saying that you won't really be able to do Rolling Like a Ball at your desk, but you can practise a few great Pilates moves to get you through your work day without leaving your desk.

CHEST EXPANSION

Sitting at a desk doesn't help our posture, but Chest Expansion can. Stand in Pilates stance (see p.60) with your back to your chair. Firm your abdomen and press your arms back until your palms are pressing lightly into the chair. Squeeze your shoulders backwards as you turn your head right, then left, then centre. Take your arms forward as you exhale. Repeat 5 times, 3 times a day.

Our days have rhythmical cycles of high energy and low energy when you'll find yourself more or less productive according to your energy levels. Exercise can give you an organic energy boost. Furthermore, on days when you simply can't fit in an entire workout, small bursts of activity can serve the body's need for regular exercise and keep you conditioned and healthy.

I have selected the following combination of moves to get you up and out of your chair, address full-body and joint mobility, as well as counter some of the negative effects of sitting at a desk with less-than-perfect posture all day long. This short routine, done one move at a time or all at once, provides core control, spinal strength and alignment, as well as upper-body conditioning.

Expand the chest as you press back towards the chair

Hug the knee tight to the body

SINGLE LEG STRETCH

This exercise is borrowed from one of Mr Pilates' disciples, Carola Trier. Begin slowly and concentrate on keeping yourself centred and strong. There is no twisting allowed.

Slide down on your chair so that your bottom is right at the front edge and your upper back is leaning against the back of the chair. Draw one knee into the chest and stretch the other leg out long. Slowly begin alternating legs, keeping your abdominals scooped (see p.61) and your elbows wide. Repeat 10 slow repetitions twice a day.

Stretch the leg parallel to the floor

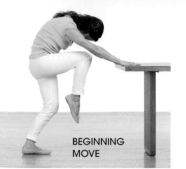

BEGINNING MOVE

STANDING KNEE STRETCHES

Mobilise and strengthen with this move from the mat. Place your hands on your desk and step back until your arms are straight. Keep your legs parallel as you lower your head and tighten your tummy. Inhale and bend one knee up towards your forehead. Now kick the leg back as you exhale, bending the supporting leg and arching your upper body up. Repeat for 10 quick stretches, then switch to the other leg and repeat.

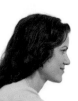

Stretch the arms long and press the palms flat

Support the core

Hold the standing leg firm

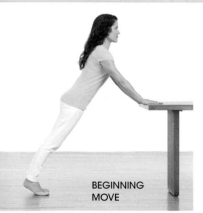

BEGINNING MOVE

PUSH-UPS

Push-Ups don't always require a floor. Just stand up from your chair and work your upper body the Pilates push-up way.

Stand tall facing your desk or table. Place your hands at the edge of your desk for support and step your feet back until you are in a straight diagonal line. Keep your arms in line with your shoulders as you bend your elbows back and bring your chest towards the desk. Straighten back out, keeping your abdomen firm. Perform 8 slow repetitions twice a day.

Pull the navel to the spine

Keep the heels lifted

Pilates for relaxation

Relaxation doesn't always mean nap time. Ideally your relaxation is balanced with an equal amount of alertness. Here is a series of exercises that promote relaxation at any time of day, along with the details of how Pilates helps you de-stress and relax fully.

General exercise helps you relax in a number of ways. As our breaths per minute increase with activity, we automatically regulate our breathing. Under normal conditions, most people breathe at less-than-optimal oxygen uptake. Since decreased oxygen is directly related to stress, tension and panic attacks, exercise can help to balance your carbon dioxide to oxygen ratio. Regular exercise also helps stabilise your hormones and greatly improves your sleep and emotional wellbeing, all of which contribute to relaxation.

Pilates uses developmental sequencing to mimic the growth process of an infant. This helps settle the nervous system as well as reorganise the musculoskeletal system. Pilates' coordinated breath and gravity-assisted moves also amplify the post-exercise relaxation effect. There are specific moves you can use to infuse your days with a little relaxation. If you have time for an end-of-day workout to help you unwind, hit the mat for a full programme. For relaxation purposes, though, eliminate the standing postures at the end.

SPINE STRETCH FORWARD I (see p.78)
Tense necks and tight backs will appreciate Spine Stretch Forward I. Take your time and breathe fully and deeply, allowing the weight of your head to pull you forward and down. Stretch long, lengthen out and just breathe.
When? Great for the evening.

DOWN STRETCH (see p.139)
Inversions and deep breathing are perfect for enhancing circulation. Down Stretch has both. As an added bonus, you'll combat rounded shoulders and lazy abdominals. When performed with energy, Down Stretch will leave you both alert and relaxed.
When? Great for the morning.

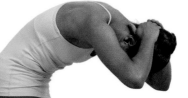

WALL CIRCLES (see p.97)

As our bone mass decreases and our spine shortens, good posture and alignment become harder to sustain. Use the wall exercises to help restore your sense of alignment and length, and to remind you what your tallest posture should feel like.

When? Great for the middle of the day.

WINDMILL (see p.92)

The perfect exercise to train your breathing technique to give you improved oxygen uptake. Work on increasing the length of your exhalation with each and every repetition to rebalance your carbon dioxide to oxygen ratio.

When? Great for the middle of the day.

STANDING SWINGS (see p.205)

Playful movement is not only rejuvenating, it's restorative. Allow your body to swing fully and freely, building a steady, easy rhythm. Focus on timing your breath with your movement. Inhale at the peak of the lift and then exhale audibly with each fall. This move shouldn't feel contrived or rigid. Just have fun!

When? Great for any time.

Pilates for better sex

If Pilates can improve your stress levels, overhaul your strength and give you better muscle tone, then there are clearly other benefits to be had. A healthy sex life is part of a balanced lifestyle and contributes to our overall wellness. Keeping fit improves sexual function and Pilates has specific applications for making your sex life that much better.

Exercise in general will improve your procreation practice in a few particular ways. The confidence you build through regular activity and exercise translates into confidence about your body. This confidence is visible to everyone and contributes to making you feel more sexually desirable. The strength and flexibility you acquire during exercise increase your sexual performance and technique – which is nothing to scoff at. Finally, regular exercise has been shown to result in an increase in sexual response in both men and women. Do I have your attention now?

So why Pilates?

Let's get specific. Working out with Pilates is part-gymnastics, part-yoga and part-calisthenics. The level of control you develop over your muscles will parlay nicely into the bedroom, where control issues sometimes get the better of us. A specific muscle known as the pubococcygeus, or PCG, is responsible for helping men sustain their lovemaking and for helping women to intensify their own experience. This PCG muscle lies within the pelvis and is part of what's known as the pelvic floor. To exercise your own pelvic floor, you should do exercises known as Kegels (see overleaf), which strengthen the PCG muscle. This muscular contraction is used in Pilates but really pays off later, when you need it most.

Secret workout

The PCG muscle works in both men and women and can be exercised in the same ways for both sexes. You can begin by imagining the feeling of stopping the flow of urine to identify this muscle. However, you shouldn't actually practise this technique while urinating as you will run the risk of infection. If you have trouble getting any sense of contraction to occur, try actively tightening the ring of muscles round the rectum. Your PCG should contract as well.

SEXERCISE
Exercises like this Thigh Stretch can make sex easier and more fun.

The psoas muscles which attach along the lumbar spine flex and extend the hips and lower back during the thrusting movements of sex.

Toning the PCG muscle (see opposite) will increase the intensity and duration of muscular contractions in the pelvic floor during sexual climax.

To build strength in this area, practise contracting your pelvic-floor muscles for a 5-second hold. Relax and repeat 5 times in a row. Increase your hold time to 10 seconds as you continue to practise. Try not to substitute other muscles like the abdominals or buttocks. To help you practise regularly, try to do a set of Kegels each time you sit down for a meal. No one will know you are secretly working out.

Breathe through it

An additional factor that gives Pilates the leg up in enhancing your sex life, is its specific breathing techniques. Learning to coordinate your breath with your movements, as we do in Pilates, has a variety of applications in the bedroom. Better breathing means you'll be sending more oxygen to the areas that are working hard during sex. Breathing techniques, such as those

KNEE STRETCHES (see p.84)
Pelvic mobility is important in keeping up with your partner.
Use Knee Stretches to focus on your range of motion in this area.
They will ensure you can go just as far one way as the other.
Good for? Sex positions on all fours.

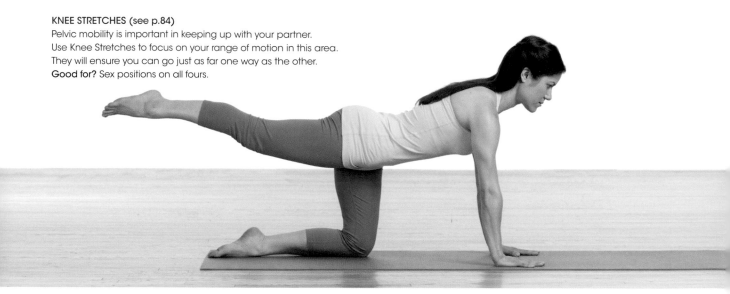

SHOULDER BRIDGE (see pp.90–91)
Strength and stamina go hand in hand between the sheets. Shoulder Bridge will strengthen your hip muscles and your glutes. No matter which direction you prefer, these muscles will serve you well.
Good for? Sex positions where your hips are raised.

employed in Tantric breathing (a method which is said to prolong sexual intercourse by enabling you to modulate your breathing), are also an option for creative sexual play.

Fostering a healthy libido

Exercise has been shown to help increase sexual response. But be careful before you lace up those sneakers. Pilates comes in way above training methods like running and cycling for maintaining a robust sex drive. In fact, intense cardio training is known to suppress the libido because a depletion of the sex hormones occurs during sustained cardio exercise. This doesn't happen with Pilates, so it's the ideal exercise choice for better sex. Use the specific exercises below in sequence or individually to develop mobility and strength in the body parts that will help make intimacy that much easier.

FRONT SPLITS (see pp.100–101)
If you want to take advantage of more than just the standard positions, you'll need to develop your flexibility and range of motion. Front Splits will really help expand your repertoire.
Good for? Sex positions where you are upright or partially supported.

THIGH STRETCH (see p.200)
Strong thigh muscles are a must for adult play. Thigh Stretch accomplishes the perfect balance of function and form – because those legs have to look good while they work!
Good for? Sex positions where you are kneeling.

Maturing with Pilates

The process of ageing begins long before we consciously experience it. The deterioration is both general and specific. The good news is that while we cannot avoid accruing more years, we can stave off many of the negative effects of ageing with exercise.

All research has demonstrated that the effects of exercise training are consistent in spite of a person's age. That means the gains you'll make in your body with regular training are similar to those a much younger person would achieve with the same training protocol. Exercise truly is the fountain of youth. And Pilates, in particular, is especially effective for the ageing physique with specific needs.

Body changes as you age

The mature adult undergoes a reduction in bone density and the skeleton becomes brittle and susceptible to injury. Contrary to popular belief, the elderly don't always fall down first and break a bone upon landing. The bone often breaks beforehand, causing a fall and compounding the problem. Along with a loss in bone density come postural changes. After the age of 40, our muscle mass also undergoes change, decreasing at the rate of one per cent per year. As for the cardiovascular system, it's no longer as effective at circulating the blood or at responding quickly to an increased workload. Blood pressure rises but metabolism slows. Memory and cognitive changes seep into the mix, depending on a host of factors. The list goes on, but what's important is what we can do about this process so that we can enjoy and extend our vitality as long as possible.

   I recommend all my mature clients establish a programme that addresses their bone density and muscle mass as well as postural alignment and breathing function. If you're not doing the programme in this book, make sure to include these elements in your training.

Why these moves?

The selection of exercises on the following pages was designed to address some of the basic issues around ageing. Once again, you're welcome to perform this sequence as a full set of exercises or simply use them one at a time, as convenient. Practise consistently, noting which exercises you find the most challenging. Focus on those moves. Consider this workout your secret weapon.

Pilates gains for mature exercisers

Here are a few reasons why Pilates is ideal for the maturing exerciser.

• It's a weight-bearing form of exercise but it's non-impact.

• Pilates develops coordination and balance through a series of complex moves.

• The breathing techniques in Pilates increase lung capacity.

• Pilates will increase body awareness and memory function through an ordered series of moves. It will also improve core and spinal strength, both of which are key for maintaining upright posture.

WARM-UP ALERT
No matter what your age
or fitness level, make sure to
warm up your body before
tackling a workout.

**STARTING
POSITION**

WALL REACH

To combat gravity and the tendency to contract the upper body and round the upper back, this simple backwards stretch is very effective.

Stand up tall with your back facing the wall. Inhale and raise your arms up overhead by your ears. Exhale and take your eyes, arms and chest up towards the ceiling, reaching for the wall behind you with your fingertips. Let your hips press forward slightly but keep lifting upwards in the chest. If you manage to make contact with the wall, walk your fingers down the wall before coming right back up. Round over your legs to finish.

First aim the tips of the fingers to the wall; as you progress, you can aim the palms to the wall

Lift the upper back and chest up high

FOOT WALK

Our feet support our bodies all day every day. Over time, the structure of our feet changes, giving rise to painful standing and walking. Keep your feet healthy and strong with this targeted foot exercise.

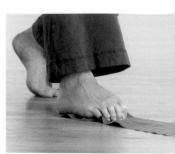

Sit comfortably with your foot placed on the edge of a small exercise band or towel. Spread the remainder of the band out long. Grip the end with your toes and curl up your arch, dragging the band in towards your heel (right, above). Release by fanning your toes (right, below) and grip the next portion of the band.

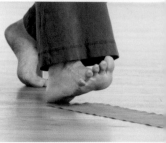

Continue until you reach the end of the band. Spread the band out to repeat again. Then switch feet.

Layer the hands on top of one knee

Stretch the band out long and flat

PILATES SQUATS

Our joints naturally stiffen over time and can limit our mobility. To keep the best possible range of motion in your ankles, knees and hips, perform this exercise regularly.

Stand with your feet parallel and hip-width apart. Hold onto the back of a chair for better balance. Keep your heels flat and bend your knees, taking your hips far back behind you. Keep your head and chest lifted. Pause at the bottom, then rise back up, bringing your upper body back as you straighten your legs. Repeat 8 times. For a challenge, try this without the chair.

Keep the chest lifted up high

Lead with your rear end as though you were about to sit down

WEIGHT SHIFTS

Balance is a key component to healthy living. Like muscles, balance is something you can easily train and improve. Use this exercise to develop your sense of space and your proprioception – your sense of your body's position in space – which will markedly improve your balance.

Stand tall with both arms stretching out to the sides and your feet in a small "V" (Pilates stance, see p.60). Take a small step to the right and try to balance on your right foot as you lift your left leg just off the floor. Keep your upper body straight. Hold for a breath, then come back to the centre on two feet. Repeat to the left. Continue switching from right to left for 10 reps. For an added challenge, place your hands on your hips.

Keep your box square (see p.62) as you shift

Extend the arms strongly to help balance

Hold firm in the supporting leg

Pilates for rehabilitation

In his book *Your Health*, Mr Pilates referred to his method as "health control". As a physical therapist myself, I can attest to Pilates' rightful place in a therapeutic setting. What I find the most valuable is the way Pilates can straddle the fence between passive, assisted rehabilitation and active, self-guided rehabilitation.

Here are a few concepts that Pilates training is known for and that are usually utilised in any effective rehabilitative setting.

MINIMUM OF MOTION
Your Pilates workout will train your body to eliminate extraneous movements when navigating from point A to point B. Since many injuries happen during transitions from one position to another, this training is extremely valuable.

MAXIMUM EFFICIENCY
When you're not fiddling around wasting energy, your movements become that much more effective and efficient. Efficient movement saves energy, allowing you to move much faster and more freely.

MIND OVER MUSCLE
Most rehabilitation makes some use of a process known as biofeedback, which trains an individual to be aware of and ultimately control his or her physiological functions such as heart rate and muscle activity. Focus and

BREAK IT DOWN
Following rehab, many of your Pilates moves will be broken down into smaller components. Swimming is one such exercise that can be reduced to smaller, focused movements.

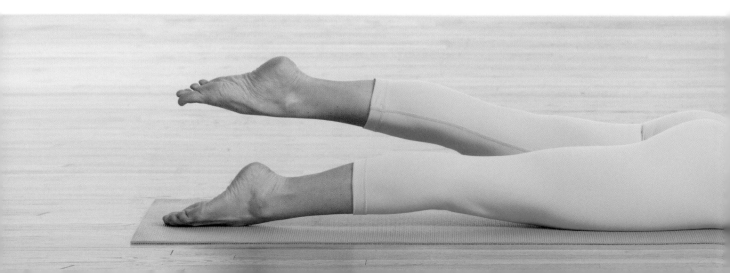

concentration (see p.42), which are key in Pilates, make a tremendous difference in the healing process. Pilates is a perfect place to practise this biofeedback process and have a dialogue with your body.

MOBILITY AND STABILITY

Anchoring one body part to free up another is the basis of human motor development. The body must learn to stabilise before it's able to mobilise. Pilates develops this practice.

Healing the body

There are many types of injuries from which you may be recovering. For limitations stemming from musculoskeletal conditions, there are steps towards recuperation that aim to restore optimal function to an injured area.

As a first step, you must always focus on restoring the complete range of motion. For example, a knee injury may leave you able to bend your knee only part of the way. The most important goal of your therapist will be to get your knee to bend fully. If you're using Pilates to supplement your rehabilitation, you may use some exercises that focus on actively bending and straightening your knees, such as Single Leg Stretch (see p.76) or Double Leg Stretch (see p.119).

The second rehabilitative stage is to regain strength. A weakened shoulder might be strengthened with a Pilates exercise like Sparklers (see p.95) and later on by more weight-bearing exercises like Push-Ups (see pp.196–7).

The last category of rehabilitation is speed. Once your injured area has acquired its original range of motion and original degree of strength, speed is the final level of training. Regardless of the exercises in your programme,

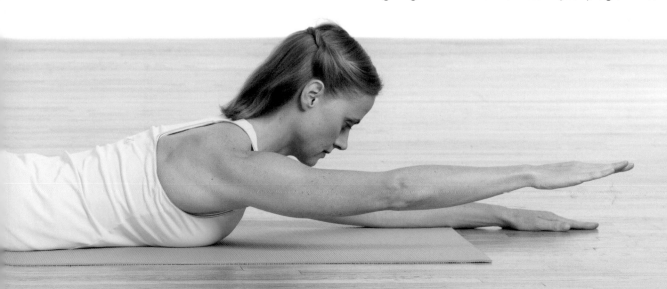

your tempo will increase and more dynamic elements will be added, such as quickly changing directions.

If you're currently in physical therapy and have the privilege of Pilates as part of that therapy, you'll probably work with the Pilates equipment and experience the resistance of working with springs. Mr Pilates originally developed his equipment in a rehabilitative setting. It was working in a hospital that actually led him to use springs to help patients who were bedridden and needed the springs to assist their weakened muscles. Springs work very differently from regular weights because they require your control and coordination in all directions. In addition, the tension applied to your muscles by the springs changes and adjusts throughout the exercise,

CENTRING (see p.68)

Moving from a stable centre (see p.44) is the best strategy for training your muscles to move freely. A more stable core actually gives the rest of your body more mobility. Use this move to reset your powerhouse (see p.61) and connect with the feeling of your centre.

Work to initiate this move from a stable centre

SWAN PREP (see p.83)

Rounded shoulders and poor posture are largely the result of gravity weighing us down all day long. Swan Prep uses gravity to push us down and then requires us to lift back up against it. This move is simple and effective for targeting the entire length of the spine.

Keep the navel lifted as you begin

making your muscles work that much harder to control their movement. If you've been discharged from rehab and have been recommended to a post-rehab exercise programme, Pilates is often the first choice.

During your rehab, you'll need to address your body as a whole as well as some of the smaller weaknesses you have that may have led to your injury in the first place. Spinal strength, core stability, gluteal strength and lower-body alignment are areas that often require attention.

Once you've begun to practise the Pilates method, you're far less likely to incur small injuries, but should an injury occur, you're more likely to have a speedy recovery. The following moves are some options for post-rehab training once you are cleared for exercise by your therapist.

WALL: STAND (see p.96)

To maintain and reinforce proper alignment while standing, Wall: Stand is a great anytime exercise. Take note of any asymmetries you may feel and work to correct them as you work against the wall.

Work to align the spine straight along the wall

TWO BY FOUR (see p.99)

Our lower limbs have a lot of potential for injury. Keeping them strong, symmetrical and aligned is key to preventing injuries in the future. Whether as a preventative or therapeutic exercise, Two by Four will help strengthen and mobilise the hips, knees, ankles and feet.

Keep the hips, knees and ankles in one long line

CHEST EXPANSION (see p.102)

Weak upper backs and tight chest muscles are a by-product of the poor posture we exhibit every day. To keep our skeletons well organised and our inner organs functioning properly, exercises like Chest Expansion are invaluable.

Work to initiate from the upper-back muscles

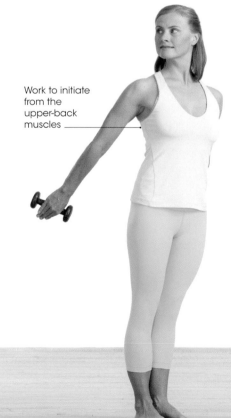

The Pilates diet

Your diet is critical to your exercise plan. My best advice to my clients is to feed their body for optimal performance. Food is just fuel and every morsel you put into your body should do something for the machine it fuels.

It's not nearly as easy as it sounds and most people struggle much more with their diet plan than they do with their exercise plan. There are a million methods and systems. Some work. Others don't. Short-term diet changes don't really do much for you in the way of permanent body shape other than confuse your system. But there are some ideas that will make a global change to your eating style. You may be surprised to see that they are some of the self-same principles that govern your Pilates practice. These principles translated to your diet can help you make permanent changes.

Pilates dietary principles

THE FIRST PRINCIPLE IS CONTROL Well, that's obvious isn't it? Control has to be present in your food choices, your serving sizes and your meal frequency. To help you execute the control principle, use the following "hand method" for serving guidelines to keep you on track with your portions:

When it says	That's about the size of
1 cup vegetables or fruit	One clenched fist
1 serving of snack food (30–60g/1–2oz)	One cupped hand
1tsp sugar	One fingertip
1tbsp oil	One thumb tip
1 serving of meat or fish (85g/3oz)	One palm
1 serving of cheese (30g/1oz)	One thumb

As well as portion control, make an effort to control the types of food you include in your diet as well as exactly when you eat and when you don't eat.

THE SECOND PRINCIPLE IS CONCENTRATION Mindless eating is the primary culprit in overeating and poor food choices. When we consciously prepare our food, we make better selections, balance our diets and become steadily healthier. Make it a practice never to eat in front of a television, computer or even while reading. Focus exclusively on your meal.

SEE, SMELL AND TASTE
Each meal is a sensory experience.
Pay attention to your meal as you eat,
taking in the aromas, textures and
variety of tastes and colours.

Concentration and diet together are a two-way street. Just as you should work to focus on your diet and eating, the foods you choose can help you to stay more alert and have better concentration. Here are a few foods considered to be food for the brain:

• **Fish** – great for brain function and a healthy heart. Aim for at least two servings of fish per week – preferably fatty fish like salmon and mackerel.

• **Nuts** – high in vitamin E, which plays a role in offsetting a decline with age in cognitive function. Enjoy up to 30g (1oz) a day of unsalted nuts!

• **Blueberries** – a super berry that's wonderful for improving learning capacity at any age. Eat a cup (225g/8oz) per day.

Be cautious about giving in to sugar and caffeine cravings. You don't need to eliminate them, but you should choose carefully where you get your boost from. Glucose in fruit and caffeine from dark chocolate are preferable to simple table sugar and coffee, both of which will give you only a temporary wake-up and leave you more tired than before.

Finally, use your skills of concentration when you feel the first signs of hunger. Pause for a moment and bring your awareness to your midsection. Ask yourself if you're truly hungry. Recall how long it's been since your last meal. Perhaps you're just thirsty. Use the scale on the right to gauge your hunger before you eat, as well as during a meal and, most importantly, after the meal is over.

How hungry are you?

A simple rating system of 1 to 10 can help you put your hunger in perspective and keep it in check.

10 = Stuffed to the point of feeling sick

5 = Comfortable, neither hungry nor full

1 = Starving, dizzy, irritable

Strive to remain between 4 and 6 throughout the day.

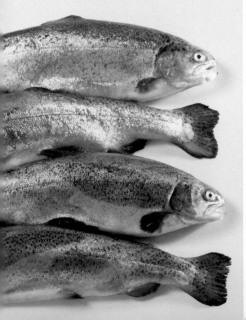

FISH
Rich in nutrients and vitamins, fish should be part of your diet at least twice a week.

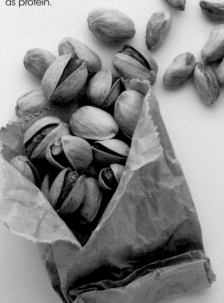

UNSALTED NUTS
A satisfying snack, nuts can provide essential fats as well as protein.

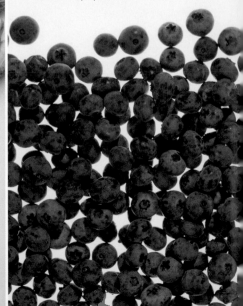

BLUEBERRIES
Known as a "superfood", blueberries should be part of every diet for their mental and physical benefits.

THE THIRD PRINCIPLE IS BREATH This final principle deserves a little extra space since it involves some complex relationships. Your senses of smell and taste both relate to your breath. Your sense of smell is triggered when you breathe in, or inhale. Your sense of taste is affected by the state of your breath and of your taste buds. You can use this knowledge to help influence your food cravings.

Let's start with those inhalations. Much research has been done on eating and food odours. The link between people's olfactory sense (their sense of smell) and their hunger has been well established. Specific aromas affect not only what you eat, but how much you eat. Newer studies show that particular smells can stimulate or suppress appetite. Strongly sweet smells can lead to feelings of hunger and then to overeating, while other smells, deemed "neutral", have the effect of curbing appetite. Below are some key tips relating to food odour that will regulate your cravings:

• **Smell the food** before you eat it.

• **Choose hot or warm food** over cold. Heating your food releases the aromas that can make the meal more satisfying.

• **Choose the most aromatic foods** that you enjoy. Heavily seasoned foods with strong aromas, such as garlic, onions and other herbs and spices, have been shown to satisfy your appetite more completely. Bland foods, on the contrary (see the next tip, below), can leave you feeling deprived.

• **Limit dairy products.** Milk and other dairy products are often so bland that they don't trigger a feeling of satisfaction in the same way as other foods. As a result, you may find yourself overeating high-calorie dairy-based foods against your better judgment.

• **Sniff a neutral food.** The odours of foods like banana, green apple, vanilla and peppermint are considered neutral. Inhaling these scents when you're feeling hungry has been shown to help to offset your appetite if you have trouble managing your serving sizes.

Next we come to the state of your breath and of your taste buds. Your tongue is a breeding ground for bacteria, which can make their way down from the nasal passages and coat your tongue. The effects of such bacteria are to dull the taste buds and cause bad breath. The practice of tongue scraping can significantly reduce bad breath but, more importantly, tongue scraping can revitalise your taste buds, making food more satisfying and reducing the urge to overeat.

Tongue scraping is not a new practice and it involves no chemicals or time-consuming processes. A simple scraper is available in any pharmacy. Be aware that simply brushing your tongue has been shown to be ineffective when compared to scraping as the bacteria are simply ground down rather than eliminated.

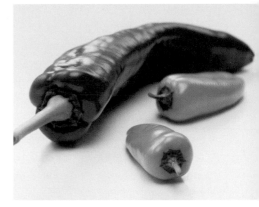

SPICE IT UP
Use seasonings and spices to create a fuller eating experience that will truly satisfy you.

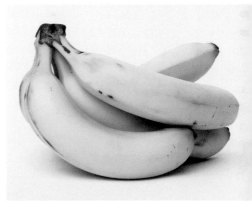

BREATHE IT IN
Taking a few breaths of neutral-smelling foods before a meal can help to prevent overeating.

Your daily eating schedule

I'm going to break rank here. Our mothers told us to eat a big breakfast and I agree that breakfast is a key meal in your day. However, after a full night's sleep, your morning meal really is breaking the fast. And if you prefer to be energised by your food rather than tax your digestive system, then eating a light breakfast is a better strategy.

So, as a rule, I recommend eating a small breakfast followed by a mid-morning snack. Your biggest meal of the day should be lunch. Think of it as a power lunch to be taken in when your body is most active and your metabolism is operating at its peak level. Dinner should be simple and completed at least two full hours before you go to bed. This eating schedule will provide you with optimal energy and a healthy routine.

We've established the principles that should determine how you eat. Here are a couple of "what to eats"! Following even a few of these guidelines will set you on a path to better health and optimal energy as well as safeguard you against many of the common pitfalls in any weight-loss programme.

- **SHOP** Choose fresh food rather than processed, pre-packaged or canned food. Frozen is the next best thing to fresh.
- **SWEETENERS** Avoid all artificial sweeteners, which simply trick your body into thinking you're ingesting real sugar. Your bloodstream will then flood with insulin and cause your blood-sugar level to drop. Then guess what happens? You're hungry again. Better to use real sugar.
- **FLUIDS** Drink a lot! Many people walk round chronically dehydrated without realising it. A constant intake of coffee and fizzy drinks that serve as diuretics cause us to lose more fluid than we're taking in. When you're dehydrated, your metabolism slows down.
- **MEALS** Fill your plate one time. Eat slowly, taking deep breaths and you'll never need to go back for seconds. Think of your main course as a side dish and go heavy on the vegetables to fill your plate.
- **TREATS** Managing a sweet tooth is a two-part strategy. First you have to define a schedule. Limiting desserts to the weekends works for some people. For others, having a small treat a day is the only way to stay motivated while on a diet. Total deprivation rarely works, so choose a plan that makes sense for you. The second thing to do is to redefine what constitutes your idea of a sweet or treat. If you can make do with a cup of blueberries and peaches drizzled with honey instead of a slice of cheesecake, then your choice is obvious. The key is to find some substitutes that satisfy you and can support your diet rather than set you back.
- **SNACKS** This is where most of us get into trouble. Snacks tend to be consumed on the go, mindlessly and throughout the day. Simply stopping

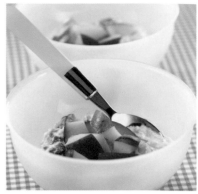

THE BIGGEST MEAL?
Change your mind about a power breakfast. Eat a light breakfast to gently wake your digestive system.

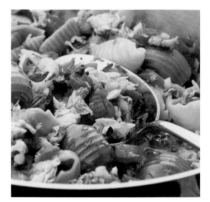

FUEL UP
Make the midday meal your largest – your metabolism is working its hardest at this time.

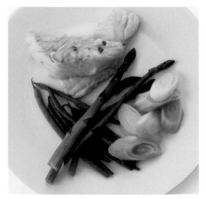

EXIT STRATEGY
You should aim to eat your last meal at least two hours before you go to bed.

all extraneous eating that isn't associated with your meals is the best way to get this bad habit under control. I do recommend 1–2 consciously planned snacks a day, but only when you've successfully eliminated the junk-food grazing that most of us fall prey to as a daily ritual.

A few easy snacks to pack ahead of time include:
• A helping of high-fibre cereal tossed in a small plastic bag
• Fresh fruit salad with a squeeze of lemon and some honey
• A small bag of almonds with up to 30g (1oz) dark chocolate
• Yogurt (without artificial sweeteners). I recommend Greek yogurt if you have access to it.

Small changes, big results?

It's very tempting to believe that one tiny change will have dramatic results when we're trying to cut calories. If you've read statistics like "cutting 32 calories a day (or 2 teaspoonfuls of sugar) can lead to a weight loss of over 1.4kg (3lb) over the course of a year" and been excited by that possibility, I have bad news for you.

The human body is ruled by the mechanism of homeostasis. This means that the body will seek to keep everything constant. It adjusts for small changes to keep things like heart rate, metabolism and, yes, weight the same.

If you were to make no other change than to cut 32 calories a day from your diet, you wouldn't experience a weight loss. Your body will adjust to burn 32 calories less per day and your weight will remain constant. If you're looking to lose weight, you must make significant changes in several areas of your food intake and calorie expenditure.

The place of cleansing and detoxing

Fresh fruit and vegetable juices are a great way to get more vitamins and minerals into your diet. One green juice a day is something I always recommend. The use of juicing to accomplish cleansing and detoxing goes through cycles of popularity. To be fair, I do support an occasional juice cleanse or fast to jump-start a healthy eating plan. However, this is the equivalent of quitting an addiction cold turkey and can be just the same as giving up coffee or cigarettes only to return after a week or a month. It's usually more prudent to eliminate unhealthy habits one at a time. Cut down on coffee before trying to eliminate it totally. Limit your desserts to weekends only before abolishing them completely. Individual changes are easier to build upon and sustain than dramatic short-term methods like juicing and fasting.

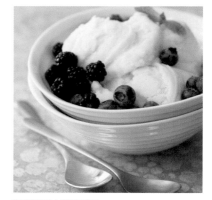

DESSERT ANYONE?
One alternative to cutting out desserts completely is to cut them in half. Share with a friend.

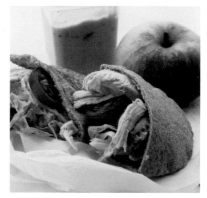

BRING ONE FROM HOME!
Snacking is a dangerous game. Bringing a homemade healthy snack can offset any junk-food binges.

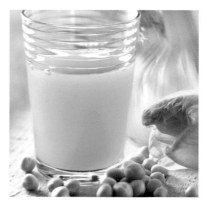

FILL 'ER UP!
Drink all day long. Water should be your first choice but also try to work a green juice into your daily diet.

Resources

Other books by Alycea Ungaro

15-MINUTE HOME WORKOUT
(Dorling Kindersley, 2010)
Written by a team of top fitness professionals, this is a complete home-fitness package, with a choice of 20 different workouts and an accompanying DVD.

15-MINUTE EVERYDAY PILATES
(Dorling Kindersley, 2008)
Perfect for when you're short of time, this book offers four 15-minute Pilates sequences, with accompanying live-action DVD.

PILATES: BODY IN MOTION
(Dorling Kindersley, 2002)
The original resource for the complete Mat repertoire including leveled workouts for beginner, intermediate and advanced exercisers.

PORTABLE PILATES™ (Pilates Center of New York, 2000)
With user-friendly illustrations, spiral binding and a 38-minute audio workout on CD, this Pilates set is a great primer to take on your travels.

Books by Joseph Pilates

From the master himself, these two resources boast the virtues of exercise and criticize our sedentary lifestyle.

RETURN TO LIFE THROUGH CONTROLOGY
(Bodymind Publishing Inc.,1998)
Learn the classic Mat exercises as demonstrated by Joseph Pilates. The complete original Mat work is presented in this historic text.

YOUR HEALTH
(Presentation Dynamics, 1998)
With recommendations ranging from dry-brushing to proper breathing, this is Mr. Pilates' essay on total wellness.

Books on nutrition

IN DEFENCE OF FOOD: AN EATER'S MANIFESTO, Michael Pollan
(Penguin, 2009)

YOUR BODY'S MANY CRIES FOR WATER, F. Batmanghelidg
(Global Health Solutions, 2008)

THE AYURVEDIC COOKBOOK,
Amadea Morningstar
(Lotus Press, 1990)

Alycea Ungaro's websites

REAL PILATES
realpilatesnyc.com
Alycea's studio in New York City, with all the equipment designed by Mr. Pilates. Real Alignment Mat, Real Pilates Sticky Socks and apparel are also available here and the website has a page offering free Pilates downloads.

REAL LIFE
alycea@alyceaungaro.com
Alycea's women-oriented website with pages dedicated to diet, fitness, entrepreneurship and business, parenting and the day-to-day challenges of women's lives.

Audio downloads by Alycea Ungaro and others

NEXTFIT
Nextfit.com
Affordable and accessible fitness by experts in a simple downloadable format with audio and video support for exercisers of all levels and abilities. Offers workouts from walking to weightlifting as well as yoga and Pilates.

IAMPLIFY
iAmplify.com
Offers a huge selection of audio and video downloads, including many for your Pilates practice.

To find an instructor worldwide

CLASSICAL PILATES
classicalpilates.net
The Worldwide Academy of Traditional Instructors lists over 1,400 professionals who completed comprehensive training with the most distinguished traditional first and second generation instructors whose training lineage comes directly from Joseph and Clara Pilates. There is also a listing of Pilates instructors worldwide.

Pilates for special populations

For men:
THE COMPLETE BOOK OF PILATES FOR MEN: THE LIFETIME PLAN FOR STRENGTH, POWER & PEAK PERFORMANCE, Daniel Lyon Jr.
(Regan Books, 2005)
Promises quick and long-term results to any man who seeks optimal fitness and a competitive edge in all aspects of his life

For pregnancy:
PILATES AND PREGNANCY: A WORKBOOK FOR BEFORE, DURING AND AFTER PREGNANCY (WITH DVD), Sarah Picot
(Picot Pilates, 2008)
This title combines an exercise workbook with a pregnancy journal, allowing you to keep track of your prenatal test results and read fun facts about your pregnancy while you stay toned, prepare your body for labour and get your figure back faster after delivery.

For post-rehab and bone health:
PILATES FOR BUFF BONES™
incorporatingmovement.com
Rebekah Rotstein is a bone-health specialist who is an author, public speaker, Pilates and post-rehab expert. She offers classes, seminars and instruction.

For Pilates professionals

PILATES PRO
pilates-pro.com
Pilates Pro is an online magazine for all Pilates professionals. It provides the industry with access to vital information, tools, services and opportunities that promote community and provide teaching and business solutions.

PILATES METHOD ALLIANCE (PMA)
pilatesmethodalliance.org
An international not-for-profit professional association for the Pilates method. The PMA's mission is to protect the public by establishing certification and continuing education standards for Pilates professionals. Find teachers internationally online.

PILATES STYLE MAGAZINE
pilatesstyle.com
Although there are dozens of fitness magazines, Pilates has relatively few references devoted to the craft. This American publication is available to overseas subscribers.

Index

Bold page numbers refer to main entries

A

abs (abdominal muscles) 57, 61
  Backward Teaser **134–5**, 149, 151
  centring **44**
  core stability 24–5
  Corkscrew **122**, 150
  Criss-Cross **164**, 210, 212, 226
  Double Straight Leg Stretch **163**, 208, 210, 212
  Footwork **162**, 208, 210, 212
  Half Roll-Up **113**, 146, 148, 150
  The Hundred **154**, 208, 210, 212
  Hundred Prep 70–71, 104, 106, 108
  Leg Pull Down **194–5**, 211, 213, 227
  Neck Peel **69**, 104, 106, 108
  Neck Pull **128**, 149, 151
  Roll-Back **72**, 104, 106, 108
  Roll-Up **73**, 106, 108
  Round Back **124**, 146, 148, 150
  Round the World I **145**, 147, 149, 151
  Teaser **190–91**, 213
  Teaser with Twist **136–7**, 151
  Ten by Ten **112**, 146, 148, 150
  Tick-Tock **82**, 106, 108
activation **61**
adrenaline 37
advanced level **153–213**
  15-minute sequence 208–9
  30-minute sequence 210–11
  45-minute sequence 212–13
ageing body **236–9**
alignment **20–21**
anchoring 57, 241
ankle problems 223
arms: Front Curls **93**, 107, 109
  problems 222–3
  Push-Ups **196–7**, 211, 213
  Side Curls **94**, 107, 109
  Sparklers **95**, 107, 109
  Tendon Stretch **182–3**, 211, 213
  Wall: Chair **98**, 105, 107, 109
  Wall: Circles **97**, 105, 107, 109, 231
  Wall Reach 238
articulation 57
"associative" phase, motor learning 34
"automative" phase, motor learning 34

B

back and spine: arching backwards 215
  C-curve **63**
  core stability 25
  Down Stretch **139**, 147, 149, 151, 230
  Flat Back **125**, 148, 150
  Half Roll-Up **113**, 146, 148, 150
  Jackknife **184–5**, 213
  Letter T **123**, 148, 150
  Mini Bridge **114**, 146, 148, 150, 226
  pain 225
  Pelvic Curl 65
  Roll-Back 72, 104, 106, 108
  Round Back **124**, 146, 148, 150
  Seal **204**, 209, 211, 213
  Semicircle **129**, 151
  Spine Stretch Forward I **78**, 106, 108, 230
  Spine Stretch Forward II **121**, 146, 148, 150
  Spine Stretch Forward III **165**, 208, 210, 212
  Spine Twist I **79**, 108
  Spine Twist II **180–81**, 211, 213
  strengthening 223
  Wall Reach 238

Backward Teaser **134–5**, 149, 151
bacteria, on tongue 247
balance: and ageing 239
  body control 28
  weight shifts 239
balls 52
bars, weighted 52, 53
baseline measurements 17
beginner level **67–109**
  15-minute sequence 104–5
  30-minute sequence 106–7
  45-minute sequence 108–9
Bicycle **186–7**, 211, 213
biofeedback 240–41
blood pressure, ageing 236
blueberries 246
body control **28–9, 42**, 48
body shape and tone **30–31**
bone density 236
Bottom Walk **80–81**, 106, 108
the box 57, **62**
brain 34
breakfast 248
breathing 13, **18–19**
  Breath-a-Cizer 46
  and diet 247
  principles of Pilates **45**, 46
  relaxation 230
  resting breathing 56
  and sex 234–5
  stress reduction 36
  tempo 56
Bridge: Mini Bridge **114**, 146, 148, 150, 226
  Shoulder Bridge **90–91**, 109, 234

C

C-curve **63**
  Spine Stretch Forward I **165**, 208, 210, 212

Spine Stretch Forward II **121**, 146, 148, 150
caffeine 246
calories 249
carbon dioxide 230
cardiovascular system, ageing 236
centring **68**, 104, 106, 108, 242
    principles of Pilates **44**, 48
Chest Expansion **102**, 107, 109, 228, 243
classes 11, **216–17**
Climb a Tree **158–9**, 210, 212
clothing 21, **52–3**
coffee 246, 249
"cognitive" stage, motor learning 34
concentration 241
    and diet 244–6
    principles of Pilates **43**, 48
confidence 232
contraction, eccentric 125
control: body control **28–9**
    diet 244
    principles of Pilates **42**, 48
Coordination **116–17**, 150
core stability 23, **24–5**, 242
Corkscrew **122**, 150
Corkscrew Overhead **168–9**, 212
cravings 246, 247
Criss-Cross **164**, 210, 212, 226
curl 57

D

daily life **220–21**
dairy products 247
desk exercises **228–9**
desserts 248, 249
detoxing 249
diet 244–9
Double Leg Kick **174–5**, 210, 212
Double Leg Stretch I **77**, 108
Double Leg Stretch II **119**, 146, 148, 150
Double Straight Leg Stretch **163**, 208, 210, 212

Down Stretch **139**, 147, 149, 151, 230
drinks 248
dumbbells 52, 53
dynamic stretching 26

E

eccentric contraction 125
efficient movement 240
Elephant 27, **142–3**, 147, 149, 151
eliminating exercises 214
ending routines 51
endorphins 36
endurance **32–3**
equipment **52–3**
"eustress" 37
exercise bands 52, 53

F

feet: Foot Walk 238
    Pilates stance 60
    socks 53
    Two by Four **99**, 107, 109, 243
firing up 57
fish 246
Flat Back **125**, 148, 150
flexibility **26–7**
flow **45**, 47
focus 49, 240–41
food cravings 246, 247
Foot Walk 238
the frame 57, **62**
Front Curls **93**, 107, 109
Front Splits **100–101**, 109, 235
fruit 246, 249

G, H

gluteal muscles **44**, 60, 61
goals 41, 223
Half Roll-Up **113**, 146, 148, 150
hand weights 52, 53
healing process 241
health benefits 16, 230
heart rate 47, 143, 240, 249
hips: Bottom Walk **80–81**, 106, 108

Hip-Ups 155, 208, 210, 212
Leg Swings: Side **144**, 149, 151
Pilates Squats 239
problems 222
Semicircle **129**, 151
Side Kicks: Rond de Jambe **188–9**, 209, 211, 213
holds 32
homeostasis 249
The Hundred 48–9, **154**, 208, 210, 212
Hundred Prep **70–71**, 104, 106, 108
hunger 246, 247
hypertrophy 22, 31

I, J

injuries 214, **240–43**
intermediate level **111–207**
    15-minute sequence 146–7
    30-minute sequence 148–9
    45-minute sequence 150–51
isometric exercise 57
Jackknife **184–5**, 213
joints, ageing 239
Jumps 47
    Standing Jumps **206–7**, 213

K

Kegel exercises 232–4
Kneeling Side Kicks **198–9**, 211, 213
knees: Knee Stretches **84**, 108, 234
    Pilates Squats 239
    problems 222, 241
    Standing Knee Stretches 229
    Two by Four **99**, 107, 109, 243

L

lateral breathing 46
lateral muscles: Mermaid **88–9**, 106, 109
    Side Bends **201**, 211, 213, 227
    Side Kicks: Double Leg Lift **86**, 109
    Standing Side Bends **103**, 105, 107, 109
leggings 52

legs: Backward Teaser **134–5**, 149, 151
Climb a Tree **158–9**, 210, 212
Corkscrew **122**, 150
Corkscrew Overhead **168–9**, 212
Criss-Cross **164**, 210, 212, 226
Double Leg Kick **174–5**, 210, 212
Double Leg Stretch I **77**
Double Leg Stretch II **119**, 146, 148, 150
Double Straight Leg Stretch **163**, 208, 210, 212
Front Splits **100–101**, 109, 235
Hip-Ups **155**, 208, 210, 212
Jackknife **184–5**, 213
Knee Stretches **84**, 234
Kneeling Side Kicks **198–9**, 211, 213
Leg Circles **74**, 104, 106, 108
Leg Pull Down **194–5**, 211, 213, 227
Leg Swings: Front **143**, 149, 151
Leg Swings: Side **144**, 149, 151
problems 215, 223
Roll-Over **156–7**, 212
Pilates Squats 239
Scissors **178–9**, 213
Side Bends **201**, 211, 213, 227
Side Kicks: Bicycle **186–7**, 211, 213
Side Kicks: Circles **132**, 147, 149, 151
Side Kicks: Double Leg Lift **86**, 109
Side Kicks: Front I **85**, 105, 106, 109
Side Kicks: Front II **130**, 147, 149, 151
Side Kicks: Inner Thighs **133**, 151
Side Kicks: Lower Lift **87**, 109
Side Kicks: Rond de Jambe **188–9**, 209, 211, 213
Side Kicks: Scissors **131**, 149, 151
Single Leg Stretch I **76**, 228
Single Leg Stretch II **118**, 146, 148, 150
Single Straight Leg Stretch **120**, 150
Standing Knee Stretches 229
Star **202–3**, 213
Teaser **190–91**, 213
Teaser with Twist **136–7**, 151
Thigh Stretch **200**, 209, 211, 213, 235

Tick-Tock **82**, 106, 108
Two by Four **99**, 107, 109, 243
Letter T **123**, 148, 150
libido 235
loading, muscles 31
"love handles" 127

M

mats 21, 52, 53
memory: ageing 236
memorising routines 35, 215
Mermaid **88–9**, 106, 109
metabolism 143, 236, 249
midline 57
mind over muscle **34–5**
mindfulness 43
minerals 249
Mini Bridge **114**, 146, 148, 150, 226
mirrors 21, 43, 52
mobility, rehabilitation 241
modifying exercises 214
motor planning, body control 28, 34
muscles: ageing 236
biofeedback 240–41
eccentric contraction 125
endurance **32–3**
flexibility **26–7**
muscle tone **30–31**
negative loading 31
straightening legs 215
strength **22–3**
working with springs 242–3
myths **12–13**

N

neck: Neck Peel **69**, 104, 106, 108
Neck Presses **64**
Neck Pull **128**, 149, 151
problems 222
negative stress 36–7
nervous system 22, 34, 230
nutrition **244–9**
nuts 246

O, P

oblique muscles: Corkscrew **122**, 150
Teaser with Twist **136–7**, 151
Twist and Reach **127**, 148, 150
Open Leg Rocker **166–7**, 210, 212
overhead exercises: Corkscrew Overhead **168–9**, 212
Hip-Ups **155**, 208, 210, 212
Jackknife **184–5**, 213
Roll-Over **156–7**, 212
Scissors **178–9**, 213
oxygen 46, 230, 234
pain, lower back 225
pants 52–3
Pelvic Curl **65**
pelvic-floor muscles: centring 44
Kegel exercises 232–4
powerhouse 61
Pilates, Joseph **8–11**, 13, 18
Pilates Squats 239
Pilates stance 57, **60**
poles, weighted 52, 53
portion sizes 244
posture **224–5**
ageing 236
stress reduction 36
powerhouse 44, 57, **61**
precision 45, 49
preparation 45
principles of Pilates 40–41, **42–9**
problems **214–15**
pubococcygeus (PCG) muscle 232
Push-Ups 22–3, **196–7**, 211, 213, 229

R

rehabilitation **240–43**
relaxation **230–31**
repetitions 51, 56
resistance 22–3, 57, 242–3
Rocking **192–3**, 213
rolling exercises: Half Roll-Up **113**, 146, 148, 150
Open Leg Rocker **166–7**, 210, 212

Roll-Back **72**, 104, 106, 108
Roll-Over **156–7**, 212
Roll-Up **73**, 106, 108
Rolling Like a Ball I **75**, 108
Rolling Like a Ball II **115**, 146, 148, 150
Rolling Like a Ball III **160–61**, 208, 210, 212
   Seal **204**, 209, 211, 213
Rond de Jambe **188–9**, 209, 211, 213
Round Back **124**, 146, 148, 150
Round the World I **145**, 147, 149, 151
Round the World II **176–7**, 209, 211, 212
routines *see* sequences

S
Saw **170–71**, 209, 210, 212
Scissors 47, 120, **131**, 149, 151, **178–9**, 213
scoop 57
Seal **204**, 209, 211, 213
Semicircle **129**, 151
sequences 47
   advanced level **208–13**
   beginner level **104–9**
   intermediate level **146–51**
   memorising 35, 215
sets 56
sex life **232–3**
shorts 52
Shoulder Bridge **90–91**, 109, 234
shoulder problems 222, 241
Side Bends **201**, 211, 213, 227
   Standing Side Bends 103, 105, 107, 109
Side Curls **94**, 107, 109
Side Kicks: Bicycle **186–7**, 211, 213
Side Kicks: Circles **132**, 147, 149, 151
Side Kicks: Double Leg Lift **86**, 109
Side Kicks: Front I **85**, 105, 106, 109
Side Kicks: Front II **130**, 147, 149, 151
Side Kicks: Inner Thighs **133**, 151
Side Kicks: Lower Lift **87**, 109
Side Kicks: Rond de Jambe **188–9**, 209, 211, 213
Side Kicks: Scissors 47, **131**, 149, 151
Side to Side **126**, 146, 148, 150

Single Leg Stretch I **76**, 108, 228
Single Leg Stretch II **118**, 146, 148, 150
Single Straight Leg Stretch **120**, 150
Sit-Ups, problems 215
sitting posture 224
skeleton: ageing 236
   posture 224
   stability **24–5**
smell, sense of 247
snacks 248–9
Snake **140–41**, 149, 151
Sparklers **95**, 107, 109
speed, rehabilitation 241–2
spine *see* back
Spine Stretch Forward I **78**, 106, 108, 230
Spine Stretch Forward II **121**, 146, 148, 150
Spine Stretch Forward III **165**, 208, 210, 212
Spine Twist I **79**, 108,
Spine Twist II **180–81**, 211, 213
Splits, Front **100–101**, 109, 235
springs 22, 242–3
stability **24–5**, 241, 242
stamina **32–3**
stance 57, **60**
Standing Jumps **206–7**, 213
Standing Knee Stretches 229
standing posture 225
Standing Rotation **60**
Standing Side Bends **103**, 105, 107, 109
Standing Swings **205**, 209, 211, 213, 231
Star **202–3**, 213
static stretching 26–7
strength **22–3**, 241
stress reduction **36–7**, 230
stretches 12, 26–7
substituting exercises 214
sugar 246, 248
Swan **172–3**, 209, 210, 212
Swan Prep **83**, 104, 106, 108, 242
sweating 13
sweeteners 248
Swimming **138**, 149, 151

T
T, Letter **123**, 148, 150
tail 57
Tantric breathing 235
taste, sense of 247
teachers 10, **216–17**
Teaser: Backward Teaser **134–5**, 149, 151
   Teaser III 41, **190–91**, 213
   Teaser with Twist **136–7**, 151
tempo 56, 242
Ten by Ten **112**, 146, 148, 150
Tendon Stretch 40, **182–3**, 211, 213
thighs: Side Kicks: Inner Thighs **133**, 151
   Thigh Stretch **200**, 209, 211, 213, 235
Tick-Tock **82**, 106, 108
tone, muscle **30–31**
transitions 45, 51
troubleshooting **214–15**
trunk, core stability **24–5**
twists: Criss-Cross **164**, 210, 212, 226
   Saw **170–71**, 209, 210, 212
   Spine Twist I **79**, 108
   Spine Twist II **180–81**, 211, 213
   Teaser with Twist **136–7**, 151
   Twist and Reach **127**, 148, 150
Two by Four **99**, 107, 109, 243

V, W, Y
vegetables 249
vitamins 249
Wall: Chair 32–3, **98**, 105, 107, 109
Wall: Circles **97**, 105, 107, 109, 231
Wall: Stand **96**, 105, 107, 109, 243
Wall Reach 238
warm-up **59–65**, 237
watchwords 16
weight loss 249
weights 52, 53
Windmill 37, **92**, 105, 107, 109, 231
work, Pilates at **228–9**
wrist problems 222–3
yoga 12

Acknowledgments

ABOUT THE AUTHOR

One of the most widely recognised and influential Pilates instructors and wellness experts, Alycea Ungaro is the founder of Real Pilates, New York City's top studio dedicated exclusively to the Pilates method.

A nutritional consultant and certified peri-natal specialist, Alycea presents workshops nationally and serves on the advisory board of *Fitness Magazine*. She has been featured in *The New York Times*, *Time* magazine, *Vogue* and *Marie Claire*, among other publications, as well as broadcast media outlets in the United States, including CBS, ABC, the TV Guide channel, NY1 News and LXTV. Alycea is a featured personality on Nextfit. com and iamplify.com, where visitors to the sites can download her signature workouts. She has released a number of popular exercise products including the patented "Real Alignment Mat", available online at www.realpilatesnyc.com. As her business and reputation continue to grow, Alycea's mission is the same as it has always been: to make the life-changing benefits of Pilates readily available to all – regardless of age, fitness level or geographic location.

Alycea Ungaro lives in New York City with her family.

AUTHOR'S ACKNOWLEDGMENTS

In 2001, Dorling Kindersley (DK) contacted me to pen their new Pilates title. I happily accepted. Their offices are in London and with me in New York, we began our long-distance relationship. The writing was done in New York and submitted via electronic mail and fax for review and editing. Our first photoshoot was held here in New York and was done the old-fashioned way. We shot the images and then reviewed the slides every night, making picture selections and identifying which moves might need re-shooting.

This year we undertook a new book and with newer technology, things were very different. Digital imaging has eliminated the need to review slides with a lightbox and a loop. Instead, we edited on-site and re-shot whatever wasn't working immediately. Edits and layouts were delivered rapid-fire and my fax machine, which was essential for my first book, was virtually obsolete. I am so grateful for the technology that continues to improve the publishing process and allows me to bring my ideas to people in the most efficient and expeditious way possible.

Technology, however, must take a back seat to the wonderful people who worked tirelessly on this enormous book. They gave their time, energy, insights and passion. An enormous thank you to the DK team for bringing me on board to create my biggest Pilates publication yet. Thanks to Peggy Vance and Penny Warren for their vision, Hilary Mandleberg for her patient and meticulous editing and Helen Murray for her attention to detail. Thanks to Anne Fisher, an Art Director who makes the most amazing "scamps" – a dying art for sure. Thanks to Wendy Bartlet, Glenda Fisher and Lisa Lanzarini for their art direction and design.

For the superb photography and a wonderful ten days together, I must thank Angela Coppola and assistant Steven Counts. For making us more glamorous than we imagined possible, Martin Pretorious. Much gratitude goes to Gillian Rosenthal, Tela Anderson and Stephanie Lanckton, Cynthia Smith, Emma Ungaro and Estelle Ungaro, who donated their bodies to the cause. For our great PR efforts, Margot Lewis and Platform Media. And many thanks to my wonderful agent of ten years, Laurie Liss of Sterling Lord Literistic.

A heartfelt thank you to those who inspired and worked with me all year long, including fitness and Pilates trainers throughout New York City. You are truly the cream of the crop. Special thanks to Nicole Meadors of Pilates Hudson and Brian Lawson of Body Architecture.

To my "real" family at Real Pilates who listened, reviewed and weighed in every step of the way – Lillian Vince, Johnny Pruitt, Jason Haro, Colette Krogol. You guys make it all possible.

Finally, a big hug and kiss to my wonderful family who I adore and for whom I ultimately do all that I do! I love you.

DK ACKNOWLEDGMENTS

DK would like to thank Alyson Silverwood for proofreading, Hilary Bird for the index, Steve Counts for assisting at the photoshoot, Martin Pretorious for hair and make-up, Dennis Seckler at NoHo Productions, Kate Meeker for editorial assistance and our wonderful models: Tela Anderson, Stephanie Lanckton, Gillian Rosenthal and Cynthia Smith.

PICTURE CREDITS

The publisher would like to thank the following for their kind permission to reproduce their photographs: (Key: a-above; b-below/bottom; c-centre; l-left; r-right; t-top)
10 Texas Woman's University: The Woman's Collection, Blagg-Huey Library. **11 Getty Images:** Michael Rougier / Time & Life Pictures. **249 Corbis:** photocuisine (br). Getty Images: FoodPix / Foodie Photography (tr)
All other images © Dorling Kindersley
For further information see: www.dkimages.com